HE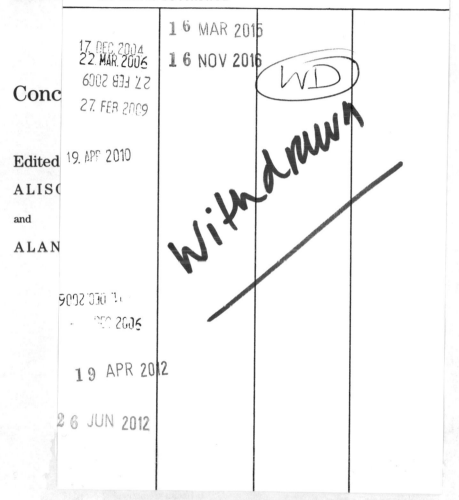

Conc

Edited

ALIS

and

ALAN

b

Blackwell Science

© 1993 by
Blackwell Science Ltd
Editorial Offices:
Osney Mead, Oxford OX2 0EL
25 John Street, London WC1N 2BL
23 Ainslie Place, Edinburgh EH3 6AJ
350 Main Street, Malden
  MA 02148 5018, USA
54 University Street, Carlton
  Victoria 3053, Australia

Other Editorial Offices:

Blackwell Wissenschafts-Verlag GmbH
  Kurfürstendamm 57
  10707 Berlin,
  Germany

  Zehetnergasse 6
  A-1140 Wien,
  Austria

First published 1993
Reprinted 1994,1995, 1997

Set by DP Photosetting, Aylesbury, Bucks
Printed and bound in Great Britain by
Hartnolls Ltd, Bodmin, Cornwall

The Blackwell Science logo is a trade mark of
Blackwell Science Ltd, registered at the
United Kingdom Trade Marks Registry

DISTRIBUTORS

Marston Book Services Ltd
PO Box 269
Abingdon
Oxon OX14 4YN
(*Orders:* Tel: 01235 465500
          Fax: 01235 465555)

USA
Blackwell Science, Inc.
Commerce Place
350 Main Street
Malden, MA 02148 5018
(*Orders:* Tel: 800 759 6102
                 617 388 8250
          Fax: 617 388 8255)

Canada
Copp Clark Professional
200 Adelaide Street, West, 3rd Floor
Toronto, Ontario M5H 1W7
(*Orders:* Tel: 416 597-1616
                 800 815-9417
          Fax: 416 597-1617)

Australia
Blackwell Science Pty Ltd
54 University Street
Carlton, Victoria 3053
(*Orders:* Tel: 03 9347-0300
          Fax: 03 9347-5001)

A catalogue record for this title
is available from the British Library
ISBN 0–632–03543–9

Library of Congress
Cataloging-in-Publication Data

Health promotion: concepts and
practice/
  edited by Alison Dines and Alan
Cribb
    p.   cm.
  Includes bibliographical references
and index
  ISBN 0-632-03543-9
  1. Health promotion. 2. Nursing
I Dines, Alison. II. Cribb, Alan
  [DNLM: 1. Health Promotion.
2. Sociology, Medical. WA 590
H43815   1993]
RT90.3.H43   1993
613.2–dc20
DNLM/DLC
for Library of Congress   93-1873
                          CIP

Contents

List of Contributors

ELIZABETH ARMSTRONG RGN, RHV, Primary Care Facilitator – Mental Health, Kensington, Chelsea and Westminster Family Health Service Authority, London.

PIPPA BAGNALL BA, RGN, Director, Queen's Nursing Institute, London.

ANN BERGEN BA, MSc, RGN, Dip N, DN Cert, Lecturer, Department of Nursing Studies, King's College, University of London.

JESSICA CORNER BSc, PhD, RGN, Onc Cert, Senior Macmillan Lecturer and Head of Academic Nursing Unit, The Royal Marsden Hospital, London.

ALAN CRIBB PhD, Lecturer in Ethics and Education, Centre for Educational Studies, King's College, University of London.

ALISON DINES BSc, MA, RGN, RHV, RHVT, FWT, PGCEA, Lecturer, Department of Nursing Studies, King's College, University of London.

DINAH GOULD BSc, MPhil, RGN, Cert Ed, Lecturer, Department of Nursing Studies, King's College, University of London.

LINDA LABUTE RGN, Dip DN, CPT, Clinical Facilitator – District Nursing, Balham Health Centre, London.

JILL MACLEOD CLARK PhD, BSc, RGN, Professor of Nursing, Department of Nursing Studies, King's College, University of London.

JANE SANDALL SRN, SCM, HVDip, BSc (Hons), MSc, Lecturer, Department of Nursing Studies, King's College, University of London.

DAVID SINES PhD, BSc (Hons), RMN, RNMH, PGCTHE, RNT, FRCN, Professor of Community Health Care Nursing, Department of Nursing and Health Visiting, University of Ulster at Jordanstown.

JENIFER WILSON-BARNETT BA, MSc, PhD, RGN, Dip N, RNT, FRCN, Professor and Head of Department of Nursing Studies, King's College, University of London.

Preface

Since the early 1980s health promotion has become ever more prominent. It has been highlighted in the Health Service reforms, it has come to be seen as an essential aspect of the work of all health professionals, and it is recognized as an important dimension of public policy. This process has also involved the inclusion of health promotion issues in curricula such as Project 2000. One of the most striking facts about this rise to prominence is the widespread disagreement as to what health promotion is or ought to be. Many people find themselves in the position of having to be in favour of something they cannot define. Often when people do have clear ideas about what is called for, they find their views are challenged or dismissed by others.

One way to respond to this disagreement is to attempt to resolve it by offering a definitive account; but others will have their own equally 'definitive' account, and we may be no further on. Another way forward, and the one we prefer, is to accept that there is something inherently contentious or contestable about the nature of health promotion, and to try to understand why this is. This is one of the aims of this book.

The book introduces the reader to a wide range of concerns in the theory and practice of health promotion. Although we hope it is accessible, we would hesitate to call it an introduction. We believe that the idea of health promotion requires a different approach.

If we want to promote health then we must have some conception of the notoriously controversial concept of *health*. In addition we have to address the many and varied approaches to the *promotion* of health. These basic ideas are somewhat general and abstract, making them inherently confusing. Some people will feel able to interpret them and 'pin them down', but in order to do so they will inevitably be seeing these ideas through their own framework of values.

In other words health promotion is not a neutral term, the meaning of which will emerge if we examine the facts for long enough. Its meaning and boundaries will be seen differently by those with different ethical and political beliefs. Perhaps the easiest way to see this is in relation to practice. Imagine yourself in any setting you like, and imagine you have been asked to promote health. Would you know what to do? If you are like us you would have a vague idea, but you would not be able to decide on what action to take without reflecting on your other beliefs and values. This is the subject of Part 1 of the book, in which we raise many questions and review a range of possible answers. Our aim, however, is to invite you to reflect on the debate, rather than to pretend that there are definitive answers.

Part 2 of the book is designed to provide insight into the opportunities and challenges that health promotion presents in practice. It is not intended to be comprehensive, but rather to represent the range of nursing practice, including the four main branches of nursing and work in both institutional and non-institutional settings.

It is possible to see each of the chapters as a self-contained whole, but we hope that you will also be interested in the relationship between the chapters. First, there is the fact that such a diverse set of themes can all be brought together under the heading of health promotion. Is this an advantage of the breadth of the term, or a sign that it is too open-ended? Second, there is an opportunity to see something of the different ways in which ideas about health promotion can be embodied in practice. Inevitably the authors, although they have much in common, have slightly different sets of values and either explicitly or implicitly place different emphases on the meaning and role of health promotion. For the foreseeable future these variations will continue. In most places they are much greater, and the disagreements far more strident, than in this book. We see all of these differences, great or small, as good. It is only by looking at many viewpoints that you can identify the strengths and weaknesses of your own position.

Acknowledgements

We would like to thank Lisa Field, for her timely advice at various stages and the following people:

Alison Dines: My parents, Edward and Marjorie Dines, for their interest and practical help. My husband, Mike Farwell, for his perpetual support, enhancing my state of well-being immeasurably!

Alan Cribb: Jacky, my family, friends, colleagues and students for their kindness.

Part One
Health Promotion: Concepts

Chapter 1
What is Health?

Introduction

'Hello, how are you?' This familiar greeting is spoken almost unthinkingly as it helps sustain the fabric of everyday life. Within it lies an implicit reference to the concept of health. Health is an abstract idea that is constantly alluded to in our conversations, but once we try to capture and define it, it melts to nothing like candyfloss on our tongue. When the Health Secretary writes, 'There is a commitment in this White Paper to the pursuit of "health" in its widest sense, both within Government and beyond' what does she mean? (Department of Health, 1992, p. 2)

This first chapter asks the question 'what is health?' There is a sense in which it is impossible to talk of promoting people's health if we are not sure what health actually is. For this reason we have made this our starting point. The following discussion explores the idea of health very broadly, considering not only official definitions of health but also how the concept is used in everyday terms. By re-examining what may sometimes be familiar territory we hope to shed some light on this difficult area.

Thinking about health

Who speaks about health?

The term 'health', it seems, is the property of everyone. We have a National Health Service, supermarkets offer us foods for 'healthy eating', religious groups proselytize for our spiritual health, psychologists encourage us to express our grief for the sake of our mental health, manufacturers persuade us to purchase the healthy option, health clubs urge us to get fit and be beautiful for a healthier life, the Government cautions against smoking which may 'seriously damage your health', and environmental groups ask us to help 'ensure the future health of our planet'. What are we to make of these various uses of the word? Do they all employ the same meaning; are some correct and others not? How are we to arbitrate between them and does it really matter?

All these varied uses of the term health demonstrate a number of observations that can be made about the concept. Although all are employing the idea of health, none actually say *what* it is. The assumption is that the meaning of the term may be taken for granted and need not be spelled out.

Why do people talk about health?

The multitude of those using 'health' suggests that it is an idea that usefully communicates about an important aspect of life. Thus people speak about health to say something about themselves, for example, 'I'm well'. Alternatively it is used to give an account of our actions, for example we may say 'I'm eating this because it's healthy', or we refer to an absence of health in explanation, such as 'he can't go, he's not so good at the moment'.

People use the idea of health as a goal in life: 'Well if you've got your health that's everything isn't it?' Or they view it as something to be missed once departed: 'These youngsters don't know how lucky they are to have their health'. For employees of various kinds, health is the substance of their work. Policy makers increasingly speak of health as a goal to be pursued through political activity, and environmental groups use the idea of health to warn us of global fragility and the need for protection and conservation.

Where is 'health' used?

We can see that health seems to pervade all areas of human existence in that it is spoken about in so many contexts. Physical health seems particularly ubiquitous, with conversations about food, drinking, exercise and smoking occurring in the workplace, at the meal table, in the supermarket and at leisure. Paradoxically medical contexts are a prime site for references to health and those caring for families and young children seem to have a particular concern with health.

Other components of health are less easily discerned, so discussions about spiritual health are more confined to intimate settings, religious groups or those facing death or bereavement. Mental health is even more elusive as a subject for discussion, until fairly recently referred to only indirectly via mental illness. Now ideas like assertiveness training, greater mental acuity and 'feeling good' through exercise and stress management have lifted the veil to some extent. Interestingly, comments about the social and emotional health of others are largely confined to gossip, while campaigners and politicians trade the goal of health used in a broad unspecified sense.

Health is an emotive concept and is spoken about in many different ways. As Backett (1990) notes, it is spoken about with feelings of guilt and smugness. It also evokes superiority and embarrassment, and can be referred to with zeal and fervour, with commitment and authority, with regret, despair and anxiety, with pleasure, celebration and hope, or with relief and prayerfully. The word health is found in colloquial talk and formal debate, and it is referred to in hushed whispered tones and broadcast persuasively to the nations.

Attempts to define health

Attempts to define health encounter a number of problems. The first centres on the fact that it tends to be taken for granted. Health seems to conform to the aphorism, 'You don't know what you've got 'til it's gone.' People do not talk a great deal about what it feels like to be healthy; they are much more articulate about what it is like to be unhealthy. Tillich (1961) recognizes how one cannot think about health without the reality and possibility of disease. Hunt *et al.* (1980, p. 282) have noted that with health it is easier to specify departures from the norm than it is to specify the norm itself. In some ways it is easier to identify certain behaviours which we evaluate to be healthy, than to define health itself. Thus we may feel the fact that we go running, play tennis or eat wholemeal bread is healthy, or that we are healthy because we have learned to be assertive, to appropriately express our emotions and enjoy some good supportive relationships. When we try to say what health *is*, we run into difficulties, or end up using glib statements that are so familiar it is difficult to hear them afresh.

Thus we may say health is not being ill or health is well-being. These two statements largely correspond with two well known definitions of health: the biomedical view that health is the absence of disease and the World Health Organization statement of 1946 that health is a 'state of complete physical, mental, and social well-being and not merely the absence of disease or infirmity' (WHO 1946). Both of these conceptions of health have certain difficulties.

Biomedical view of health

Let us first examine the biomedical view that health is the absence of disease. Intuitively this view has considerable appeal and indeed research into lay health beliefs supports the idea that a great many people do indeed conceive of health like this (Blaxter, 1987; Calnan, 1987; Williams, 1983). One problem occurs however when we consider the example of a person who has a disease but to whom we might also wish to apply the label 'healthy'. A woman with multiple sclerosis who has come to terms with her condition and is leading a full and productive life within certain limitations might be viewed by some, including herself, as healthy. A man dying with bowel cancer who peacefully approaches his own death with the support of his family, might be said to have a very healthy approach despite the fact that his life is coming to an end. Conversely, someone who rarely feels happy, who is anxious, worried and lonely, although not suffering from an identifiable disease, may not be viewed as entirely healthy. It seems therefore that the biomedical conception would label some people as diseased whom we might wish to label healthy, and others healthy whom we might wish to label diseased in some sense.

Another objection to the 'absence of disease' approach is that it is too narrow. Are we to accept that all people in the world who do not have a disease are enjoying a healthy existence? What about people wrongly imprisoned, whole populations who lurch from one day's survival scratched from the earth to the next? Are these people healthy? In the sense that they are free from disease they are, but in the sense of enjoying a flourishing existence or a sense of well-being they may not be healthy.

The limitation of the biomedical definition of health is the assumption that health is the mirror image of disease, when many people would argue that health is much more than that. The idea that disease is the opposite of health may fail to give a full picture. Issues such as poverty and injustice may also need to be taken into account when considering the converse of health. If, however, we split apart the term disease, to become *dis-ease*, then a broader conception of health may indeed be the absence of dis-ease. This of course is much more akin to the World Health Organization's definition.

Weaknesses of the World Health Organization's view

There are a number of weaknesses in equating health with complete mental, physical and social well-being, which in some measure echo in reverse those levied at the biomedical conception. A complete state of well-being appears too idealistic. In this view can anyone be healthy? Are we to disregard a significant number of people who, though not enjoying a perfect life, certainly 'don't have too much to complain about'? Are these people really not enjoying some measure of health? Alternatively, if someone was to be in a state of complete well-being what would they be like? The idea of such a state seems somehow to smack of some goody-goody, an unblemished, faultless person whom the majority of us might feel too uncomfortable to know.

If we suppose for a moment that such a state might exist, how does this fit in with the capriciousness of life itself? Can time deprive a person of his health as he ages, or deprive a child of his health as he develops? What part may outside circumstances play in influencing someone's health? When such factors are taken into account we begin to see a state where perhaps only young men and women in their 20s and 30s, at the peak of their physical prime and living in situations of material comfort, are viewed as healthy. Health becomes a very transient state in such a conception. Indeed, what about the rashness of youth and the wisdom of old age? Is the latter maturity in mental, social or even spiritual health to be demeaned in the face of physical prowess? Many people would wish to see acknowledgement that it is possible to be healthy in old age.

The final criticism that needs addressing when considering the World Health Organization's view, is its failure to consider all the facets of health. Many people would feel that no mention of a person's spiritual or emotional health is a serious flaw. The list may be expanded indefinitely depending on one's understanding of the human condition.

The same person may view health in different ways

We have so far demonstrated the difficulty encountered when attempting to define health. The concept is so hard to articulate one feels one is grappling with an enormity which both definitions discussed above provide some insight towards, although neither is sufficient. Indeed this idea itself may provide us with a very useful way of thinking about health. Seedhouse (1986, p. 7) has suggested that health means different things to different people. It may be more helpful to say simply that health means different things to people. In other words human beings operate with a number of conceptions of health at the same time. As Stainton Rogers (1991) has suggested, people are 'proficient weavers of stories', selecting from a number of options open to them as they give an account of something. We render human beings and the concept of health a disservice if we think health may be captured either in the statement 'health is not being ill' or 'health is well-being', or that human beings permanently choose either one of these as their mental picture. The fascinating truth may lie nearer to the idea that health may be viewed in many different ways by the same person, and that individuals shift, without difficulty or explanation, from one notion to the next, in a highly skilled process of selection, creation and articulation.

The idea that health may be a concept that can be defined in a number of different ways – all of which have equal validity – places it in an unusual position. It is difficult to think of many other abstract ideas which have, for example, both a restricted and broad meaning, which may without explanation be called on and discarded in communication. If we think of the idea of freedom, this may be conceived narrowly as freedom from restraint or interference, or much more broadly as a situation where people are only truly free to live their lives to the full when certain fundamental conditions are met. These might include a fair system of government, justice within the legal system, adequate education and sufficient food and water. The difference between these two senses of freedom and the two senses of health, however, lies in the fact that communication about freedom would not generally slip from one conception to the other without considerable challenge and questioning.

Health as a 'means'

An interesting question following from this is whether it is even beneficial to try and define health any more closely. The process of attempting to delineate health, even if not wholly successful, may be a useful way to discovering more about the concept itself. Seedhouse's writing reflects a significant shift in the debate about health, and his ideas are worth exploring. Both the biomedical view of health and the World Health Organization definition see 'health' as an end. It is either a state where disease is absent or one of well-being. However, Seedhouse in the title of his book *Health: the foundations for achievement* sees health as a means (Seedhouse, 1986). He equates health with the foundations for achievement. Achievement itself thus becomes the goal. This is an interesting development and is in line with more recent World Health Organization work which sees health not as the object of living but as a resource for everyday life (Nutbeam, 1986, p. 113).

This shift to 'means' has the advantage of refocusing attention towards determinants of health in the real world. In so doing, debates about the nature of health are rescued from an ivory tower and potentially have a tangible impact. For those concerned to promote health, this is a considerable advantage. We can immediately see that if people are to achieve in life, they need, for example, an adequate food intake, a certain level of education, relationships with other human beings and housing of some sort. These will be the foundations in their life.

Another way of thinking about these foundations is to see them as the determinants of health. A person's health will be determined by many things, for example, contact with infection, genetic factors, level of nutrition, access to health care, financial resources, race, class, smoking, drinking and exercise habits and exposure to hazards in the environment.

The purpose and nature of health

A difficulty with this shift to 'means' and not 'ends', however, is that we now understand more about what health is *for*, but perhaps less about what *it is*. In other words, from Seedhouse's title *Health: the foundations for achievement*, we know more about the purpose of health but possibly less about its nature. If we think of other abstract concepts for a moment, we can see that both purpose and nature are needed to aid our understanding. If we think of the idea of love as possibly being similar to the abstract idea of health, we can say something about what love is and what it is for, although both are obviously open to a great deal of debate. We might say love is a feeling experienced by one person about another person, characterised by tenderness, concern and passion. When we come to ask 'What is love for?' the question sounds strange and has a metaphysical quality. We might answer as a sociologist and say, 'Love serves to cement society together'; or we might answer from a religious perspective and say, 'Love shows us something of the nature of God'. By looking at questions of nature and purpose in this way, we can see that both provide insights into the idea of love and each tells us something more about love.

If we consider another abstract idea like democracy, again we can ask what is democracy and what is it for? In a similar fashion to the idea of love, democracy is something that has been debated for centuries. We might say democracy is a system of government where power is shared between many people. We might consider the purpose of a democracy to be the provision of a just and fair system of government, or we might feel the purpose of a democracy is to provide a smoke screen for a covert elite to continue unchallenged. Once again we can see how questions of nature and purpose provide different insights into a concept impinging here, for example, on political science.

If we return to the concept of health: Seedhouse's equating of health with foundations for achievement informs us of the purpose of health but somehow tells us less about its nature. As we can see from the analysis of love and democracy, this gives us only a partial view.

At another stage in his writing Seedhouse does appear to be speaking about the nature of health when he writes:

'a person's optimum state of health is equivalent to the state of the set of conditions which fulfil or enable a person to work to fulfil his or her realistic chosen and biological potentials. Some of these conditions are of the highest importance for all people. Others are variable dependent upon individual abilities and circumstances.'

Seedhouse (1986, p. 61)

The difficulty with this conception of the nature of health is that health as a determinate concept in its own right almost seems to disappear. Health is simply the sum of these other parts or conditions, but no greater than that. Thus the state of health is an index of a person's class position, financial situation, dietary habits and so on, but no more. Health seems to have become merely a shorthand way of expressing the accumulation of these other factors. The synergy is lost and the idea of speaking about health as an end in itself or in a determinate fashion, at times, becomes problematic. This seems to fly in the face of part of our intuitive understanding of health and something of its popular use.

It may be possible to take Seedhouse's idea of 'the achievement of personal potential' (Seedhouse, 1986, p. 63) out of context, and use it as an indicator which signifies when a person is in a state of health. The idea of personal potential is akin in some ways to the broad view of health of the World Health Organization. To some extent the idea of the achievement of personal potential as a hallmark of health is affected by the same flaws as the World Health Organization's conception of health. Thus it is possible to argue that no one can ever be identified as enjoying a state of health using this measure because no one individual ever achieves his potential. In life we are constantly confronted by decisions which demand that we take one path or another; to say yes to one option is to say no to another. As a simple example, a gifted sportsman has the potential to reach the heights in both soccer and cricket, but his choice to pursue a career in football means he fails to reach his potential in the other sport.

To return to Seedhouse's conception of the achievement of personal potential, he adds a qualification which rescues the idea from this criticism. He writes of a person working to 'fulfil his or her realistic *chosen* and biological potentials' (Seedhouse, 1986, p. 61). The idea of choice answers the difficulty discussed above. The mention of chosen potential however does assume a self-conscious act. This might be at variance with people's experience in life of 'drifting into things' which they later find suited them and are fulfilling. Thus a child raised in a musical family might never consciously choose to develop his musical talent, though he achieves his personal potential in a very similar fashion to a similarly gifted person who has made a *conscious* choice. Taken to its logical conclusion, Seedhouse's insistence on the achievement of *chosen* potentials, if used to signify a state of health, might unwittingly exclude people who fulfil their potential in an equally satisfying way although not in such a consciously chosen fashion.

The qualification of realistic chosen and biological potentials also introduces another difficulty: the mention of *realistic* potentials. It is possible to imagine that some people have very low expectations of the realistic potential of life, given the constraining circumstances in which they find themselves. The realistic, and even chosen potential of a severely malnourished child might be to die, given the absence of any possibility of life-sustaining help. This appears to match the criteria set by Seedhouse as the goal of health work, but seems to be the very converse of indicating a healthy state as popularly conceived. Seedhouse it should be noted does acknowledge this difficulty with the idea of the achievement of personal potential (Seedhouse, 1986, p. 72).

Another difficulty with the idea of achievement of personal potential is its emphasis on achievement. In the West we have a very achievement orientated society. Other cultures are less concerned with achievement and more concerned with being. Is it possible to disregard the latter as signifying a state of unhealthiness? Paradoxically, many would see our own constant striving for achievement as demonstrating a greater sense of dis- ease. Tied in with this is the question of whether a person who has all the necessary foundations for achievement at his disposal, but who chooses not to realise his potential, is to be regarded as unhealthy? If people are denied such freedom of choice, a vision emerges of what some would regard as a sick society.

Defining health

Even if attempts to define health ultimately prove futile in providing a water-tight definition, the consideration itself may be enlightening and the end product a workable approximation of the concept of health. For this reason we now explore how health might be defined.

Health is a concept used to describe the state of a living organism. It says something about the functioning of the organism, and whether it is deemed to be within normal limits. If the organism's functioning is considered abnormal it may be described as unhealthy or ill or diseased. Thus a person's pancreas may not be functioning correctly and the person may develop diabetes. Not all abnormal functioning, however, is directly relevant to health and disease. For example, some people would say a bank robber is unusual and therefore abnormal. But it is usual to describe such a person as 'bad' rather than 'mad', a criminal rather than mentally ill. Others might, for example, search for something in the criminal's past to help explain his present anti-social behaviour, thus exonerating him of blame and responsibility to some degree, and viewing him in a health – disease framework rather than a criminal one. The boundary line between morality and health is therefore blurred at the edges.

Health does not refer to normality alone because something may be normal to a situation or society but not be viewed as healthy; for example, everyone may have influenza or smoke and this may be seen as unhealthy. Health therefore also embodies a value judgement about the desirability of the state or its 'goodness'. This value judgement of desirability or 'goodness' is not made in an aesthetic or moral sense. We may not like someone picking their nose or dyeing their hair orange, but we would not normally say it was unhealthy. We might deem it unhealthy if we were concerned about the spread of infection or the health risks of hair colorants. Similarly we may not approve of stealing but we would not usually say this was unhealthy, unless we were concerned with societal health or we felt a mental health problem was leading to shop-lifting or other forms of theft. The sense in which we see health as a desirable state is in the measure to which the behaviour – belief being discussed is actually believed to contribute to normal, ideal, ordered or typical functioning in a socio-biological sense, or a richer quality of life in some metaphysical sense.

Health may merely refer to an organism functioning in a normal fashion, or it may embody something much broader in which the organism is not merely 'getting by' or surviving, but partaking of some quality in life, some richness, some sense of well-being. The latter seems to be different from the former, in one sense broader, embodying a positive component and not merely the absence of disease, and in another sense narrower, focusing upon mental or social health with less emphasis on physical health.

Relative and dynamic nature of health

Throughout the discussion so far, certain conceptions and indicators of health have been criticized as being too idealistic. Downie *et al.* (1990) offer an interesting approach to this difficulty when they suggest that health is not an absolute concept but a relative one. Thus health promotion might be more concerned to enable people to better their health than attain a specified level of health approaching perfection.

Earlier we mentioned two conceptions of health. The first view saw health as a state where an organism is functioning within normal limits, and the second extended this to a state where an organism is enjoying a measure of quality in life or well-being. Two cautions need to be sounded in relation to these ideas. The first concerns the focus on a state and the second concerns the focus on an organism. The term state implies a fairly static situation which changes little over time. In many ways health does not conform to this. A person may be enjoying a state of mental well-being one day, but then suffer a bereavement the next day which leads to a period of depression. Alternatively a person might feel a high level of self-esteem and belonging through enjoying working and living in a particular area. If he or she is then made redundant and feels forced to move to find a job, this level of social health may be diminished for a time. For this reason it may be more useful to emphasize the dynamic nature of health, rather than see it as a state which is relatively unchanging.

Planetary health

The second difficulty with the earlier discussion about the two concepts of health concerns the focus on organisms. Within the past decade attention has been drawn to the health of the planet as a whole and the dependence of the human race on this global form of health. A focus on organisms rather neglects this dimension, unless we see the planet as one large organism. Recently a suggestion has been made, in keeping with planetary health, that the concept of health should be broadened to a sustainable state. One writer who supports this view is King (1990). He suggests adapting the World Health Organization definition of health to become a *sustainable* state of complete physical, mental, and social well-being, and not merely the absence of disease or infirmity. He argues that sustainable health enables the individual to live out his normal lifespan and, more importantly, the means of achieving this must be consistent with the health and existence of future communities. A crucial difference with this view of health therefore is an extension of the concept *beyond* the death of the individual, to a concern with future populations. If this is accepted, the implications are far reaching and at times unpalatable. A healthy lifestyle becomes one that is lived in a sustainable relationship with the ecosystem, eschewing profligacy in the present so as not to compromise the health of future generations. King sees such a lifestyle in the industrial northern hemisphere of the world as involving consumption control, with:

'intensive energy conservation, fewer unnecessary journeys, more public transport, fewer, smaller, slower cars, warmer clothes and

colder rooms. It also means much more recycling and a more environmentally friendly diet with more joules to the hectare.'

(King, 1990)

In the underdeveloped southern hemisphere, with the global population growing by 1 million every four days, this leads to the disturbing
question of whether measures such as oral rehydration should be
introduced on a public health scale, increasing, as King suggests, the
man-years of human misery, ultimately from starvation. The idea of
planetary health and a concern with the sustainability of the ecosystem
does appear in earlier writing from the WHO. Nutbeam (1986, p. 114)
refers to a socio-ecological concept of health recognizing the inextricable
link between people and their environment. The idea assumes more
urgency as we learn more of the breakdown of the 'buffering action of the
sky and the sea to accept waste products' (*The Lancet*, 1990, p. 659).

Health as normal functioning related to health as well-being

The relationship between the two concepts of health as normal functioning and well-being is an interesting one. It might be possible to
suggest that normal functioning, in the sense of ordered or ideal functioning, is the same as well-being. A person who is functioning without
disorder in a sociobiological sense might be free of disease, feel good,
positive and enthusiastic, experience a sense of joy and peace, feel
physically fit, enjoy his relationships with family and friends and feel he
has a part to play in the world. This picture, however, may seem far
removed from most people's everyday experience. It is also possible to
suggest that a person who is functioning normally in a typical or statistical sense might sometimes attain these heights of experience but not
always.

Other writers have wondered whether well-being is really part of the
concept of health at all, or whether it is merely a related concept closely
allied to health but distinct from it. This is an important question because
it will influence what health promotors feel is their sphere of activity.
Downie (1990, p. 6) writes: 'While the concepts of health and well-being
overlap they are distinct and cannot be combined into one concept'. The
idea that health and well-being overlap but are distinct is interesting.
Downie appears to hold this view for two reasons.

First, because health as the absence of disease and as well-being
cannot be seen as opposite poles on a linear scale. We have already
mentioned this in our discussion of the weaknesses of the biomedical
conception of health. We noted that we might wish to label as healthy, in

some sense, a terminally ill man with bowel cancer who is peacefully approaching his own death, with the support of his family. Conversely, someone who rarely feels happy, who is anxious, worried and lonely, although not suffering from an identifiable disease, may not be viewed as entirely healthy.

Downie takes this as evidence that the absence of disease and well-being may not be two components of a single concept. If, however, the idea of a linear scale is discarded and replaced by viewing health as a spectrum, then it might be possible to envisage the absence of disease and the presence of well-being united within the concept of health. The key difference here is the recognition of the various dimensions of health, so that the patient with bowel cancer enjoys poor physical health but good spiritual, mental, social and emotional health. In contrast, the anxious lonely person has good physical health but poor emotional, social, spiritual and mental health.

In Fig. 1.1 the spectrum of health is composed of various dimensions, each themselves made up of segments which may be viewed as healthy, or unhealthy or ill. Thus a person may have degrees of healthiness and illness at the same time, enjoying a measure of well-being while *at the same time* not entirely free of disease. If we see well-being and the absence of disease as opposite poles on a linear scale this would not be

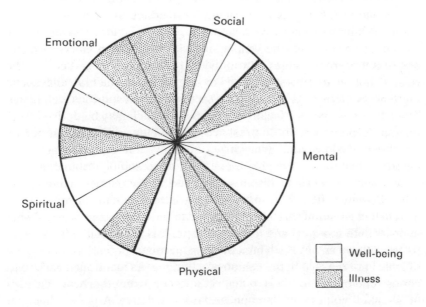

Fig. 1.1 The well-being – illness spectrum (adapted from Dines, 1993).

possible, for in order to be in a state of well-being a person must then *also* be in a state where disease is absent. If the idea of a spectrum is accepted, well-being and the presence of disease can co-exist along the various dimensions of spiritual, emotional, social, mental and physical health. Such a state is illustrated in Fig. 1.1.

The second reason Downie (1990) feels health and well-being are related but separate, is that well-being includes broader issues more akin to concepts such as happiness, enjoyment and welfare, rather than a 'glow of health' that he more comfortably equates with health. Downie's hesitancy here seems principally to be due to a concern that health promotion alone, and by implication health workers alone, must be concerned with health. As soon as the concept of health as well-being expands into spheres such as enhancing welfare through better housing, or links to a sense of satisfaction derived from some creative work, he seems reluctant to take the argument to its logical conclusion. When such difficulties are faced it might be more appropriate to recognize that health workers do not have the monopoly on health as well-being, rather than to narrow the conception of health to those parts of well-being that more naturally fall within the scope of health services and health workers as we know them. In contrast to Downie, it is logically possible to see the dimensions of the health enterprise as far wider ranging and involving many who would not necessarily see themselves as involved with health promotion.

Elsewhere Downie *et al.* (1990) do not appear to adhere to this view of health and well-being as overlapping but distinct concepts, when they distinguish between negative health and positive health. The latter they see as 'compromising true well-being (with its roots in empowerment, and of considerable value to the individual and society) together with the related notion of fitness, and as having physical, mental and social ingredients'. True well-being is thus separated from spurious well-being. The latter they see as a feeling of well-being which may be derived from hedonistic activities. In contrast true well-being is brought about by acquiring lifeskills and achieving autonomy and empowerment. To empower people is to enable them to develop self-determination, self government, a sense of responsibility and to encourage self-development. Downie *et al.* (1990) summarize the latter as 'being all you can be'.

Taken in isolation this 'being all you can be' conception of well-being appears both too ideal and too pessimistic. It is not possible for anyone to 'be all they can be'. Each human being has many potentials, only some of which are realised in the course of a lifetime. As mentioned earlier, to choose one option in life is to neglect another. In another way, the idea of 'being all you can be' is unnecessarily restrictive. A person living in damp accommodation with insufficient money for food might be said to be 'being all they can be' within the limited constraints of their existence, but this would hardly be a state of well-being. For these reasons the summary statement of 'being all you can be' seems rather inadequate as a way of conveying the idea of acquiring lifeskills and achieving autonomy or empowerment.

Fitness, wholism and well-being

It is interesting to see that Downie *et al.* (1990) separate out fitness for special mention as a related notion in their conception of well-being. The assumption is that fitness cannot be subsumed under the absence of disease or under well-being, but deserves special status as a related notion. If we return to the idea of health as concerned with an organism functioning within normal limits, it might be possible to view fitness as part of this. Equally, if normality refers to functioning in an orderly fashion, possibly with some implicit reference to an ideal state for the organism, then fitness might be part of such a conception.

Alternatively, if well being has a physical component, then once again it is hard to conceive of an organism, for example a human being, in a state of positive physical well-being without enjoying a measure of fitness. It is unclear therefore how helpful it is to isolate fitness from well-being, or whether it is sufficient to see well-being as an embracing concept incorporating, for example, fitness.

One last concern about this conception of well-being as '... having physical, mental and social ingredients', is the neglect of all the dimensions of health (Downie, Fyfe and Tannahill, 1990). These include emotional and spiritual elements which many people would feel embody well-being even more vividly than social, mental and physical components.

The concept of health is sometimes linked to the concept of wholism. There are a number of elements to this: a concern with the 'whole' of people, the 'whole' of society, the 'whole' dimensions of health and the 'whole' of health determinants. Thus in this view, body, mind, spirit and emotions act as a unified whole in a state of health.

The interdependency of human beings is also emphasized, with the recognition that we are 'part of one another' in some sense. Importance is additionally placed on all the various dimensions of health and all their determinants, so mental and physical health would receive equal weighting, as would the need for clean air and adequate shelter. The philosophy of wholism espouses the virtue of completeness or unbrokenness. It emphasizes the synergistic nature of health, man and society, where all the component parts act together in synergy creating a whole which is greater than the sum of its parts. This is sometimes known as a gestalt view.

The wholistic view of health is useful in highlighting the interactive nature of the constituent parts of health, human beings and the world, the importance of which we seem to have rediscovered in the West in recent decades. People are increasingly aware of the mind–body link in matters of health and illness, of the 'global village' in which we live and of the way in which people may be prone to respiratory disease through not only exposure to infection but also damp living conditions and air pollution. Wholism also alludes to a balance between these various parts; balance is an idea which some writers link to the concept of health. This stresses the importance of equilibrium in life.

It is this concern with balances that causes some people to label a person who is fanatical about fitness or diet as unhealthy, due to a lack of balance between the quest for these things and the rest of the person's life. Similarly an acquisitive society accruing too great a share of the world's resources, although benefiting its own citizens might be viewed as unhealthy because of the inequality it perpetuates. A society's pre-occupation with some dimensions of health and some determinants of health to the detriment of others might be the subject of similar criticisms; for example in our own society we have focused until recently almost exclusively on physical health in our health care systems, and health workers have attended to risk factors of disease in contrast to other determinants of health like poverty or inadequate housing.

Conclusion

This chapter began by recognizing the difficulty of trying to capture and define a concept as complex as health. The discussion has followed a journey through some difficult territory and we are left with a picture that it is impossible to express in a few sentences. We noted earlier that the government has committed itself to the pursuit of health 'in its widest sense' (Department of Health, 1992). The question of whether this really means eliminating disease or enhancing well-being or includes a concern with sustaining the planet for future generations, is open to debate. The uncertainty surrounding the meaning of health makes the work of the health promoter a difficult task. The situation is not eased by an equal confusion surrounding the meaning of health promotion, which we consider in the next chapter.

References

Backett, K. (1990) Studying Health in Families: A Qualitative Approach. In: *Readings in Medical Sociology* (eds S. Cunningham-Burley & N. McKeganey), pp. 57–84. Tavistock/Routledge, London.

Blaxter, M. (1987) Attitudes to Health. In *The Health and Lifestyle Survey* (eds B. Cox, M. Blaxter, A.L.J. Buckle, N.P. Fenner, J.F. Golding, M. Gore, F.A. Huppery, J. Nickson, M. Roth, J. Stark, M.E.J. Wadsworth and M. Whichelow. Health Promotion Trust, London.

Calnan, M. (1987). *Health and Illness: the Lay Perspective.* Tavistock, London.

Department of Health (1992) *The Health of the Nation.* HMSO, London.

Dines, A. (1993) Copyrighted illustration entitled 'Health as a spectrum' in *Fundamental Skills and Concepts in Patient Care,* by Lewis and Timby, Chapter 3, The concept of health (1992). Chapman and Hall, London.

Downie, R.S. (1990) Ethics in health education: an introduction. In *Ethics in Health Education.* (ed. S. Doxiadis) pp. 3–13. John Wiley and Sons Ltd, Chichester.

Downie, R.S., Fyfe, C. & Tannahill, A. (1990) *Health Promotion Models and Values.* Oxford University Press, Oxford.

Hunt, S.M., McKenna, S.P., McEwan, J., Williams, J., Papp, E. (1981) The Nottingham health profile: subjective health status and medical consultations. *Social science and medicine,* **15A**, 3(1), 221–9.

King, M. (1990) Health is a sustainable state. *The Lancet,* **336**. (15 Sept. 1990) pp. 664–7.

The Lancet (1990) editorial. **336**. (15 Sept) pp. 659–60.

Nutbeam, D. (1986) Health promotion glossary. *Health Promotion.* **1**. (1) 113–26.

Seedhouse, D. (1986) *Health: The Foundations for Achievement.* John Wiley and Sons Ltd, Chichester.

Stainton Rogers, W. (1991) *Explaining Health and Illness. An Exploration of Diversity.* Harvester Wheatsheaf, London.

Tillich, P. (1961) The meaning of health. *Perspectives in biology and medicine.* 5, p. 92.

Williams, R. (1983) Concepts of health: An analysis of lay logic. *Sociology.* 17, (2 May, 1983), pp. 185–205.

WHO (1946) *Constitution.* World Health Organization, New York.

Further reading

Department of Health (1992) *The Health of the Nation.* HMSO, London.

King, M. (1990) Health is a sustainable state. *The Lancet,* **336** (15 Sept.) 664–7.

Seedhouse, D. (1986) *Health: The Foundations for Achievement.* John Wiley and Sons Ltd, Chichester.

Stainton Rogers, W. (1991) *Explaining Health and Illness. An Exploration of Diversity.* Harvester Wheatsheaf, London.

Chapter 2
What is Health Promotion?

The question, 'what is health promotion?' may be approached in a number of ways. The answer may be prescriptive, setting out the parameters health promotion ought to adhere to, or it may focus on reality, offering a descriptive account of present practice. Very little attempt has been made to address this question from first principles, asking what meaning do the terms enjoy in our language? Here we examine the nature of health promotion from such a perspective, exploring the logical geography of health promotion and critically evaluating the assumptions and arguments embodied within it.

Health promotion from first principles

An examination of the concept of health promotion from first principles raises a number of questions, including what is health, what do we mean by promotion, and as a corollary, what then is health promotion? Can health be promoted, what does this assume and what are the implications?

Meanings, assumptions and implications

The concept of health has been reviewed in depth in Chapter 1. The question 'what is health?' is an issue that has exercised thinkers to a considerable degree. Responses have varied from the minimalist biomedical view, where health is the absence of disease, to the broad-ranging concept by the World Health Organization, articulated in 1946: 'a complete state of physical, mental and emotional well-being and not merely the absence of disease or infirmity'. WHO (1946). More recently Seedhouse (1986) has shifted the debate from viewing health as an end to interpreting health as a means: 'health is the foundations for achievement'. The antonyms of disease and illness are illuminating when considering the concept of health, in the case of disease highlighting the presence or absence of a pernicious entity or process that may be labelled, and in the case of illness focusing on the subjective negative or positive experience of the individual concerned.

Answers to the question 'what is promotion?' are more straightforward than those surrounding health. Two senses of the term emerge from an examination of language. The first derives from salesmanship: there may be a promotion for a particular product, whereby through audio-visual means and persuasive argument customers are encouraged to purchase what is on offer. In this way to promote is to sell, to put forward and to place in the forefront of attention. The second interpretation emanates from the workplace: a person may be promoted to a new position. Here promotion concerns raising to a higher level. The antonyms of promotion in these senses are similarly worthy of exploration. To denigrate refers to lowering the worth or esteem attributed to something. To depress or demote signifies pressing or holding down or lowering. These might loosely be seen to correspond to the two nuances of promotion considered above.

Combining the insights from the conceptual analysis of health and promotion produces a novel way of approaching the question 'what is health promotion?' Health promotion becomes placing the absence of disease, foundations for achievement and well-being in the forefront of attention. Alternatively it becomes raising well-being and strengthening foundations so achievement may be at a higher level, or eliminating more disease so that the human state remaining exists at a higher level. Conversely health promotion will minimize those circumstances that hold down well-being or denigrate the importance of foundations for achievement. Similarly it will place in the forefront of attention circumstances which minimize pernicious disease and will seek to raise subjective evaluations of well-being from the negative to the positive.

If this conception is accepted, can health be so promoted? Teasing out certain key phrases from the above analysis, it is possible to measure them against real life experience. Is there a sense in which it is possible to raise well-being to a higher level? To use one illustration, if part of well-being is being valued by others, then utilizing therapeutic techniques to enable people to relate to each other with greater satisfaction may be one way of achieving this. Similarly, is it possible to eliminate disease so that the human condition remaining exists at a higher level? Immunisation programmes to eliminate measles have such an objective in mind and are partially successful in realizing it. Circumstances that hold down well-being, such as ignorance or want may also be minimized, for example through the creation of the welfare policies in Great Britain in the post Second World War period.

It seems in certain circumstances, therefore, that there is a sense in which health may be promoted. More generally, health promotion assumes we have the necessary knowledge, will and resources needed to promote health. All of these preconditions are open to some dispute. We know smoking to be harmful to health but we do not fully understand the most effective ways of helping people to stop smoking. Our knowledge of some determinants of health is only partial and this similarly constrains health promotion.

Health promotion presupposes the necessary will to work for its goals. Individuals and societies may at times choose or, of necessity, value other things above health. People may enjoy eating butter and continue consuming it despite a knowledge of possible harm, valuing pleasure above health. A society may suffer a high level of unemployment and feel unable to ban alcohol advertising with its possible detrimental effect on such a major employer. Health promotion presupposes the existence of resources both financial and human. If women are the chief food preparers in the home, while at the same time having employment outside, the time for 'healthy' food preparation may not realistically be available within the family. An African country may be acutely aware of the need for clean water and education about AIDS, but it may have the financial resources for neither.

If the preconditions of health promotion are met, the implications of the process are worth exploration. Raising well-being to a higher level and engaging in activities to eliminate disease imply broad ranging work involving different sectors of society. If a link between unemployment and depression is accepted, then work to raise well-being in this sense might, for example, draw on employers, central and local government and financial institutions, and possibly international agencies and the unemployed themselves. Similarly, attempts to eliminate a disease such as coronary heart disease might extend beyond the public and the so-called health services to include the catering trade, food manufacturers, government financial policies and food legislation. Health promotion work implies the need for constant investment if the status quo is to be maintained and advancement made. Health is a dynamic state necessitating infinite resources. A person may have sufficient clean water today but the work has to be recommenced tomorrow if health is to be safeguarded.

At times the output of health promotion may be difficult to measure or identify. This is particularly true when focusing on well-being beyond the absence of a particular disease. Establishing a method to tap health, which by nature is subjective, dynamic, elusive and composed of complex facets which may act in synergy, is highly problematical.

Health promotion work implies some conception of the good life. The notion of well-being embodies certain values. Is a person in a state of well-being when he engages in shop lifting 'to make ends meet'? Does a society enjoy a high level of well-being if some of its members experience high mortality and morbidity rates in contrast to others? These questions of value will be explored in greater depth in later chapters.

A sometimes unforeseen implication of health promotion is that, far from reducing demand, for example for health services, it has the potential to generate greater demand. If a person receives no food and subsequently dies through malnutrition then he no longer makes any demands for health promoting resources. If however the same person receives food and recovers from his malnutrition, he may then at a later time require health promotion resources to eliminate for example, typhoid infection, a demand that would not have been made had he previously died. Weighed into this equation must of course be the benefits that the continued life of the person has generated for himself and society. But health promotion does not only imply benefits.

The boundaries of health promotion

An interesting consequence of this discussion is that all of life might be seen as health promoting. Are there any well-being depressing activities? Is the human condition solely concerned with strengthening foundations for achievement and eliminating disease? It is possible to identify activities where the purpose is not the elimination of disease; a solicitor involved with commercial law may have little connection with disease elimination. It is more difficult to identify activities which are not concerned with strengthening the foundations for achievement. A teacher may feel his work imparts skills which predispose to achievement. A bricklayer may not immediately identify with this goal, but if adequate housing is a prerequisite to achievement he may be seen to play his part. A terrorist may be seen as a destructive force opposed to others' peaceful achievement, but he may view his own work as a direct challenge to the nature of the foundations valued by a particular society or what signifies achievement within it. In his own terms he strengthens the foundations for achievement.

Are there any well-being depressing activities? Is there anything that falls beyond the remit of health promotion or well-being raising? One might think of unpleasant occupations such as working in a sewage disposal centre or down a coalmine, but both contribute to the well-being of society through the production of sanitation and energy, and through employment they benefit the individual. Does war depress well-being or might even that be subsumed under what may appear to be a malignant conception of health promotion?

Certainly for the individuals harmed through death and destruction it would seem undoubtedly the antithesis of health promotion, but if one considers the motivation of the participants the situation becomes more complex. If one enters a war to eliminate a tyrannical ruler it might be possible to suggest that such an activity becomes health promoting, strengthening the foundations for achievement in a safer world once the deed is done. Such an absurd conception of health promotion demands some boundaries before it becomes a phrase with so broad an interpretation as to be totally meaningless.

Health promotion in the literature

It is possible to identify two kinds of questions in the literature which discusses the nature of health promotion. First, there are questions about what might be called the domain of health promotion, i.e. 'what range of activities or processes does health promotion refer to?' Second, there are questions about the value of health promotion, i.e. 'what principles or values are being advocated when we are asked to adopt a health promotion perspective?'. Every time someone talks about the need for health promotion or stresses its importance, they must have some picture of the answers to both these sorts of question. But as we have seen, these are very difficult issues to get clear. Although it is a somewhat artificial way to proceed, we will consider the two questions in turn. First, we consider some attempts to define boundaries.

Health promotion and disease prevention

The term health promotion is of relatively recent origin, coming to prominence in the 1980s. The literature regarding the nature of health promotion is at times vague and contradictory and no clear cut understanding emerges from a review. Tones (1985) recognizes the possibility of examining the nature of health promotion from first principles, when he writes: 'At one level of analysis the notion of Health Promotion must logically refer to *any activity designed to foster health*'.

Dennis *et al.* (1982) appear to adopt a similar conception when suggesting 'health promotion covers *all aspects of those activities that seek to improve the health status of individuals and communities*'.

Most other work in this area rejects this approach in favour of a more prescriptive analysis. Such writing discusses the nature of health promotion outlining what criteria health promotion *ought* to adhere to, both by delineating boundaries and adopting certain values. Tones acknowledges this second approach when he writes: 'Nonetheless the term is not necessarily used to describe a whole range of activities but rather as a particular category of operations having some specific virtue'.

Nutbeam (1986) in his health promotion glossary distinguishes health promotion from disease prevention, the two being separate but complementary activities which overlap in a variety of situations and circumstances. He writes:

'Disease prevention is essentially an activity in the medical field dealing with individuals or particularly defined groups at risk. It aims to conserve health. It does not represent a positive conception of health that moves ahead, but is concerned with maintaining the status quo. Health promotion on the other hand, starts out with the whole population in the context of their everyday lives, not selected individuals or groups. Its goal is to enhance health.'

An even more distinct separation between health promotion and disease prevention is made the US Department of Health, Education and Welfare (1978, 1979, 1980):

'Disease prevention begins with a threat to health – a disease or environmental hazard – and seeks to protect as many people as possible from the harmful consequences of that threat. Health promotion begins with people who are basically healthy and seeks the development of community and individual measures which can help them to develop lifestyles that can maintain and enhance their state of well-being.'

In the above logical analysis, disease prevention was taken to be part of health promotion. Health promotion became, among other things, 'placing the absence of disease in the forefront of attention', 'eliminating more disease so that the human state remaining exists at a higher level' and 'placing in the forefront of attention circumstances that minimize pernicious disease entities'. How can these views be reconciled, if at all?

At one level perhaps a sleight of hand has occurred in the initial analysis; perhaps disease prevention and health promotion are distinct both in positive and negative orientation, audience and direction. The provision of sports facilities might be an example of health promotion, while immunisation may be an example of disease prevention.

The distinction is less clear cut, however, if it is recognized that exercise not only promotes positive health but also helps reduce the likelihood of heart disease. Is taking exercise therefore a means of health promotion or disease prevention? The distinction between conserving health and enhancing health as identified by Nutbeam (1986) will not bear close examination. The threat to health from lack of exercise precipitating disease is hard to distinguish at times from the US Department of Health, Education and Welfare's (1979) alternative conception of lifestyles that maintain and enhance well-being. It is possible to suggest that if health is to be enhanced, this must include its conservation; similarly if well-being is to be maintained, protection against any threats to health will be a crucial part of the process.

Some authors do not make a separation between health promotion and disease prevention: 'Health promotion comprises efforts to enhance positive health and prevent ill-health, through the overlapping spheres of health education, prevention and health protection' (Downie *et al.* 1990). What these writers do exclude from their definition of health promotion, however, is work focused on curative, high technology or acute health services. The rationale they give for this is twofold: first, a broad-ranging definition of health promotion is useless and unhelpful with its blurred boundaries, and second, and more importantly, such delineation is necessary to stimulate investment in alternative, previously neglected areas, as opposed to the powerful established areas of health service provision and other spheres (Downie *et al.*, 1990; Tannahill, 1985).

Two challenges may be levied at this view. The quest for clarity in the boundaries surrounding health promotion may itself be a futile exercise distracting attention from more important value questions. This argument is to be addressed in more detail later in this chapter. The second challenge questions the need to divorce health promotion from curative medicine in order to attract funds and redress the inequity in health service provision and other spheres. There *is* an important need for funding alternative ways to achieve 'health for all'. It may indeed be more difficult to articulate this message clearly if there is a risk of confusion with established areas, and powerful challenges have to be met. To suggest however that these are sufficient reasons to redefine health promotion work, excluding the contribution of traditional health services to the 'health of all' is ill-founded. Is it really possible to speak of raising well-being to a higher level without acknowledging the importance of eliminating disease? Of course health promotion cannot be reduced to this alone, but to attempt to separate it entirely risks creating an illogical conception which lacks intuitive credibility. French (1990) is one of the few authors who explicitly includes disease management, along with disease prevention, health education, and the politics of health in his typology of health promotion.

Health promotion as everything or nothing

The rejection of a very broad-ranging conception of health promotion by Downie *et al.* (1990), on the grounds that it is unhelpful and useless, is worthy of further exploration. In the analysis of health promotion in the earlier part of this chapter we explored the question of whether all of life can be seen as health promoting. A malignant conception of health promotion appeared to emerge, capable of subsuming such divergent experiences as war, terrorism and sewage disposal under the banners of foundations of achievement and raising well-being. Such an absurd conception of health promotion seems to demand some boundaries before it becomes a phrase with so broad an interpretation as to be totally meaningless.

Others have foreseen this difficulty. The World Health Organization discussion document on the concepts and principles of health promotion (1986) suggests: 'Given these basic principles an almost unlimited list of issues for health promotion could be generated: food policy, housing, smoking, coping skills, social networks'. Later they allude to a difficulty this may create: 'There is a possibility that health will be viewed as the ultimate goal incorporating all life.

Tones (1985) envisages that health promotion officers might be involved with health education, legal, fiscal and environmental change and promoting positive health, creating 'the awesome prospect of a super being who is charged with the task of promoting everything worthwhile anywhere using all available means'.

How might one sensibly begin to delineate the limits of health promotion, or is this ultimately an impossible task? The World Health Organization also attempts to separate health promotion from medical care: 'Health promotion is basically an activity in the health and social fields, and not a medical service'. Later in the same document health promotion is discussed in relation to other areas which are therefore implicitly denoted as belonging outside its remit although having some influence on it: 'Policy development in health promotion can then be related and integrated with policy in other sectors such as work, housing, social services and primary health care'. Without scrutinizing it too closely, perhaps this provides a useful working approach to delimiting the boundaries of health promotion; i.e. health promotion could be used to stand for those activities or processes which promote health but which fall outside the domain of other recognized personal, social, public or health services. The danger of this approach seems to be that health promotion may come to stand for nothing when all of the other areas and processes are taken away. It seems we can easily slide from a view of health promotion as all-encompassing to one in which it disappears completely.

'Health education plus'

In many people's minds health promotion and health education are inextricably linked. Some of the time they are almost used as synonyms.

Yet there is nearly always an implicit assumption that health promotion is a wider ranging term, that it is health education 'plus'.

Health education is one route to the improvement of people's health. It encompasses all those activities which aim to provide health via learning of one kind or another. Health promotion, partly by contrast, is seen as a general term which encompasses health education and all the other routes to health. The view that health promotion is 'health education plus' is relatively clear and useful, and it has the additional advantage of reflecting one of the origins of the term, i.e. the growing realization on the part of health educators that information giving or even lifeskills teaching (or self-empowerment) need to be supplemented by the promotion of health change through social or environmental measures.

As we have seen, Tannahill's model of health promotion relies on the 'health education plus' account. He sees three elements in health promotion: health education, preventive medicine and health protection. This model is helpful but it also conceals an important problem. It tells us some of the things that fall within the domain of health promotion but it does not tell us about the boundaries of the domain. We return to the problem of boundaries: is there any activity or process the enhancement or diminution of which might not amount to health promotion?

This puzzle about the boundaries of health promotion comes about because of the vast number and the diversity of the determinants of health and illness (see Chapter 1). Even if we confine ourselves to identifying the causes of disease or disability, this entails an apparently endless catalogue of biological, environmental and social factors. Action on any set of these factors would potentially amount to health promotion.

One symptom of this puzzle is the fact that health professionals often have differing and sometimes strongly held opinions about the meaning of health promotion. For example, some see it as one facet of health care, that part in which professionals through strategies such as education and professional-client partnerships seek to enable people to take more control over their lives and health; whereas others see health care as merely one facet of health promotion, the latter embracing all of the political, economic and environmental determinants of health, and the former referring to only that part in which professionals and patients interact. In this way it is possible for individuals to operate with very different, and partly conflicting, personal models of health promotion and this can be a real obstacle to effective communication.

The discussion about health promotion 'values' below (and in the following chapters) will throw some light on the puzzle about boundaries but in the meantime it may be helpful to say more about the causes of the confusion.

To this end it is useful to compare the term health promotion with other general terms like 'teaching' or 'nursing'. At first sight there seem to be exactly the same boundary problems with these terms; it would be very difficult to draw agreed parameters around their use. But there are two related reasons why the problem is worse with health promotion. First, it is possible to start to get a picture of the scope of these more established terms by looking at the institutional settings and professional roles with which they are associated. Although teachers are not the only people who 'teach', and nurses are not the only people who 'nurse', it makes perfectly good sense to look at these roles and the variety of settings in which they are practised, in order to understand their meaning. Health promotion does not belong to any institutional setting or professional role.

Second, these other terms (and the same is true of health care) normally suggest agents or agencies who perform activities of some kind. When we hear them we think of nurses, or other carers, etc. Yet this is not necessarily the case with health promotion; this could just as easily refer to abstract unplanned processes, or to the side-effects of the actions of individuals or groups who would never dream of calling themselves health promoters. In some senses a change of climate may be health promoting. This helps to explain why the term is inherently vague. There is no specific domain of activities, or group of people, tied by tradition or even recent convention to the business of health promotion. It has no obvious boundaries and hence discussions which attempt to delimit its domain are liable to run into trouble.

Health promotion as an advocacy of values

Fortunately it is still possible to turn to the second of the two questions with which we began looking at the literature, i.e. what principles or values are being advocated when we are asked to adopt a health promotion perspective? This is the question which the WHO (1986a) principles of health promotion are designed to answer:

(1) Health promotion involves the population as a whole.
(2) Health promotion is directed towards action on the determinants or causes of health.
(3) Health promotion combines diverse but complementary methods or approaches.
(4) Health promotion aims particularly at effective and concrete public participation.
(5) Health professionals have an important role in nurturing and enabling health promotion.

These principles are, in effect, a call for a change of perspective or attitude in those who have an interest in improving health. The first two principles amount to a plea for a wholistic perspective. Rather than focusing only on those who are sick or at risk of contracting specific diseases, policy makers and practitioners should consider all people, and all the causes and aspects of health. The last two principles above stress that health is not the exclusive province of 'experts' and make the values of partnership, public participation and collaboration integral to health promotion. Once more a change of perspective, or a 'gestalt switch', is advocated. Health workers should cease to see themselves working *on* the public or doing things *to* them, but instead see themselves acting *with* the public. Instead of prescribing they should be listening and enabling. Taken all together these principles are about giving people the internal and external resources 'to increase control over, and to improve, their health' (WHO, 1986a), to make healthier lifestyles easier to lead.

The Ottawa Charter for Health Promotion (World Health Organization 1986b) further elaborates some of these principles, and sets out the broad areas of strategy needed to implement them. The Charter lists social justice and equity as prerequisites for the improvement of health: 'Health promotion focuses on achieving equity in health. Health promotion action aims at reducing differences in current health status and ensuring equal opportunities and resources to enable all people to achieve their fullest health potential'. Although this clearly moves health promotion into the moral and political realm, the drafters of the charter identified unequal opportunities and poor environments as key causes of disease and ill-health, and hence as central to the health promotion agenda. This is consistent with most of the influential work about inequalities in the UK (to be discussed in Chapter 3), but it serves to emphasize the value-laden nature of this and many other descriptions of health promotion. According to this literature, health promotion is not just the improvement of health but is the improvement of health in ways which accord with a set of values (wholism, participation, equity) and an ethos of co-operation and collaboration.

The Charter is also interesting for its list of what health promotion action means:

(1) Build healthy public policy.
(2) Create supportive environments.
(3) Strengthen community action.
(4) Develop personal skills.
(5) Reorient health services.

A fuller version of this is given in the Appendix. A wide range of strategies is advocated, and the language with which this is done helps to provide an answer to the boundary puzzle discussed earlier. Health promotion is not seen as a new range of activities, or as a sub-set of existing activities, but as a method of harnessing any and all activities and processes which go on in society. Everyone, including health workers, is asked to become self-conscious about the way any policy or practice, whatever it is ostensibly aimed at, affects health. This is perhaps the central feature of the 'gestalt switch' that is called for. As we achieve this level of self-consciousness and it is built into our public and private conversations, then, it is argued, we have a basis on which to plan and press for health improvements.

A good example of this call for a change of outlook in the Charter is the need to 'build healthy public policy', to put health 'on the agenda of policy makers in all sectors and at all levels, directing them to be aware of the health consequences of their decisions and to accept their responsibilities for health'. Whether we are dealing with transport, housing, employment or taxation policies at national or local levels we can and should be asking about their health implications alongside their other purposes or consequences. It makes no sense to pretend that health issues or policies can be considered in isolation from the complex network in which they are enmeshed. The same is true of the environment which pays no respect to boundaries between sectors whether private or public, regional or national. All aspects of our living and working environment are potentially health sustaining or diminishing.

The third and fourth health promotion strategies more closely correspond with traditional health education models which focus on the importance of internal rather than external resources, i.e. the potential for nurturing and empowering people, both as groups and as individuals, so that they are better able to define and take control of their own health needs. Yet again certain values, such as the creation of and respect for personal autonomy, are taken to be intrinsic to health promotion.

Getting a clear sense of this whole set of values, along with the demand to reorient health services in the light of these values, is arguably the best step for health professionals seeking to understand what is meant by health promotion. The insistence on the development and dissemination of health promotion within the health services can be interpreted as a shorthand reminder of the constant need to re-examine the value basis of health care. What are the aims of the institutions, settings and individuals that make it up? How responsive are services to the diversity and specificity of individual's needs and demands, and how ready to enter into partnership? How far should health care accept the social context in which it operates, or how far should it seek to target inequity?

For many people health promotion provides a neat encapsulating phrase to stand for the advocacy of a range of values most of which most people subscribe to, at least in principle, but which can easily become obscured or forgotten in the pressures of practice. To have this label can be useful in agenda-setting and policy making. From this point of view the central question is not 'what is the domain of health promotion?' but 'is *this* being done in a health promoting way?', and this is a question that can be asked about any and every example of practice, not merely those which are clearly aimed at disease prevention or health education.

References

Dennis, J., Draper, P., Holland, S., Shipster, P., Speller, V. & Sunter, J. (1982) Prevention is possible if you try. *The Health Services*, 26 Nov. 1982 p. 13.

Downie, R.S., Fyfe, C. & Tannahill, A. (1990) *Health Promotion Models and Values*. Oxford University Press, Oxford.

French, J. (1990) Boundaries and horizons, the role of health education within health promotion. *Health Education Journal*, **49**, (1).

Nutbeam, D. (1986) Health promotion glossary. *Health Promotion*, **1** (1) 113–26.

Seedhouse, D. (1986) *Health: The Foundations for Achievement*. John Wiley and Sons Ltd, Chichester.

Tannahill, A. (1985) What is health promotion? *Health Education Journal*, **44** (4), 167–8.

Tones, K. (1985). Health promotion – a new panacea? *Journal of the Institute of Health Education*, **23** (1) 16–21.

US Department of Health, Education and Welfare (1978) *Disease Prevention and Health Promotion*. Washington DC.

US Department of Health, Education and Welfare (1979) *Healthy People*. Washington DC.

US Department of Health, Education and Welfare (1980) *Promoting Health/ Preventing Disease: Objectives for the Nation*. Washington DC.

WHO (1946) *Constitution* World Health Organization, New York.

WHO (1986a) A discussion document on the concept and principles of health promotion. *Health Promotion* **1** (1) 73–76.

WHO (1986b) *Ottawa Charter for Health Promotion*. World Health Organization & Health and Welfare, Ontario, Canada.

Further Reading

Bunton, R. & Macdonald, G. (Eds) (1992) *Health Promotion. Disciplines and Diversity*. Routledge, London.

Downie, R.S., Fyfe, C. & Tannahill, A. (1990) *Health Promotion Models and Values.* Oxford University Press, Oxford.

Ewles, L. & Simnett, I. (1992) *Promoting Health: A Practical Guide,* 2nd edn. Scutari Press, London.

Tones, K. Tilford, S., Robinson, Y. (1990) *Health education, Effectiveness and Efficiency.* Chapman and Hall, London.

Wilson Barnett, J. & Macleod Clark, J. (Eds) (1993) *Research in Health Promotion and Nursing.* Macmillan Press, London.

WHO (1986) A discussion document on the concept and principles of health promotion. *Health Promotion* **1** (1) 73–76.

WHO (1986) *Ottawa Charter for Health Promotion.* World Health Organization & Health and Welfare, Ontario, Canada.

Chapter 3
Social and Political Issues in Health Promotion

It is clear by now that health and health promotion can only be understood as part of the social contexts in which they exist. A crucial dimension of these contexts is politics. The common association of politics with party politics, or with the activities of politicians, makes it easy to assume that there is a part of health promotion that relates to politics and a part that does not. Something like this might be read into some of the pictures of health promotion discussed in Chapter 2 which, for example, distinguish between the 'politics of health' on the one hand and 'disease management' on the other (French, 1990).

One of the aims of this chapter is to show that this is not the case; that in a sense everything is political. A better starting point is not to think of politics as a domain but as a way of seeing the world. This is the same as the approach we took with health promotion. We can try to understand the world of politics but in addition we must try to understand health promotion *politically*. One way of beginning this is to reflect on the notion of inequalities in health.

Inequalities in health

As we have already seen, the very idea of health promotion is associated with calls for equity and the reduction of inequalities in health. In some ways this is uncontroversial because many health care workers have long held similar attitudes to the provision of health care. To a large extent these attitudes are built into the organization and culture of institutions like the NHS. First, we expect there to be equal access to treatment on the basis of need. Second, we accept that those with greater needs deserve more time and attention than those who are relatively well. Thus there is a tendency for those involved in health promotion, and for many others, to endorse equity goals as a matter of course. This position might be summarized as follows:

(1) There are inequalities in health.
(2) They are a bad thing.
(3) Someone (e.g. the state, professionals) ought to do something about them.
(4) Health promotion is (part of) the answer.

Although this is crude it captures the dominant theme in the politics of health promotion. It is always worth taking a closer, and sceptical, look at dominant positions. Is it true that there are inequalities in health, and if so are they always bad? Ought we to do everything in our power to eliminate them, and therefore is every attempt at health promotion justified? Exploring these questions will help to shed light on the social and political dimensions of health promotion.

There are inequalities in health – is this true? Some people have more disease than others and some people die earlier than others. It is only necessary to look at one's family and friends to see that this is the case. So there are certainly *differences* in health experiences, but is this the same as inequalities? If your aunt lives longer than your mother is this an inequality in health? It seems odd to say so; after all we expect there to be some variations in health and longevity. It seems that we restrict the idea of inequalities to systematic patterns rather than individual variations. Further, we normally restrict this idea to patterns which are somehow 'caused' by social factors rather than being a result of chance or biology. This is not a simple or clear distinction. A variation that is apparently natural might have come about because of a social inequality in the past, perhaps in a previous generation. Also, if we could undo some supposedly natural variations by targeting resources or by technical intervention, but we fail to do so, then it could be argued that we have responsibility for their continued existence. In both these cases we might therefore choose to say that these are inequalities.

The variations dealt with in *The Black Report* and *The Health Divide* (Townsend *et al.*, 1988) show wide class variations in health. These reports analysed data on mortality and morbidity and taken together they demonstrated that health variations by class appear to have increased rather than diminished over the 60 years following 1930, the period during which the health service was established and developed. These analyses have confirmed what many have long known, that an individual's chance of a long and healthy life depends in large measure on his or her social class. There are fairly steep social class gradients for all the major diseases, which means that roughly speaking the better off you are the less chance you have of suffering from them. Other work in this area suggests that we can expect to see these variations increasing in the future (Smith *et al.*, 1990). It is also possible to document similar variations with respect to race, gender and other personal and social factors.

So it seems that there are inequalities in health, and it might appear perverse to even question the idea. But it is important to do so to bring out the ambiguity in the concept of inequality. There is both a descriptive and a normative (or value-based) aspect to inequality, and it is very easy to fudge the two together or to slide carelessly from the former to the latter. At a descriptive level a difference or variation is an inequality in the sense that two measures are not mathematically equal. But inequality is also connected to ideas like unfairness or injustice, and in this normative sense to say something is an inequality is to make a value judgement about it, to say that it is bad or wrong. When the health promotion literature refers to inequalities in health, both senses are normally being drawn on: 'There are inequalities in health' means 'There are inequalities in health and they are a bad thing'. But should we move without hesitation from one to the other? This is a difficult question and before we can answer it we need to take a detour.

Making sense of society

These two different senses of inequality indicate something of the difficulty of making sense of society. We talk about social and political matters in very different sorts of ways; we apply different frameworks and employ different kinds of language. The distinction between a descriptive and a normative account of society (although it is problematic at a deeper level) is a helpful place to start. It seems sensible to distinguish the facts from the values. It looks as if some practitioners and academics are concerned more with one than the other. For example, an epidemiologist who collects data to identify patterns of disease and aims at explaining their causes and control seems to be primarily concerned with facts, whereas a policy maker who is aiming to bring about a 'better' (more healthy, more equitable) society must have a clear sense of values, of what *ought* to be as well as what is. The former, it might be said, is practising science and the latter is engaged in ethics and politics.

Hence it is possible to see the descriptive and normative senses of inequality as representing two different ways of making sense of society, and the widespread discussion of inequalities in health is occurring at the intersection of these different frameworks. Inequalities are of epidemiological interest; they focus our minds on the causes of ill-health and on what factors are responsible for the variations. They give us some indication of the scope for preventive health care. If it was possible to improve all the life circumstances of the most disadvantaged to the level of the most advantaged, what health gains could be expected? In addition, inequalities are of moral and political importance. Should we accept that there are advantaged and disadvantaged, or ought we to feel obliged to do something about it? If we feel it is right to work for greater equality what are the limits on this, what price (e.g. in freedom) is worth paying?

The study of politics has to encompass all these sorts of questions. Indeed, many people make a distinction between two branches of the study of politics – political science and political philosophy – the former focusing on describing and explaining the facts of politics, and the latter concentrating on evaluating forms of organization and asking 'what is a good society?'. To put it crudely, we can see politics as about *power*, and understanding how power works; or we can see politics as about *justice*, and trying to understand what social arrangements are just.

Traditionally politics as a subject has been associated with the government of states and with society in the sense of whole societies. Of course there are tremendously important issues of power and justice which relate to this level of analysis, but political processes and related issues can be analysed at every level of human organization. We can take an interest in the politics of health promotion at two levels at least. First, there is the question of the way in which society in general is supportive of health, and the role of the state and public policy in promoting health. Second, there is the question of the immediate social and professional context in which we work. This context will embody power relations between professionals, and between professionals and client groups, and will also give rise to debate about what is acceptable and fair. Some of these are debates on the ethics of health care (see Chapter 4) but most of them also have a political dimension.

In the next section we look at some of the explanations of ill-health and the role of social and political explanations. Following that we will consider the relationship between the promotion of health and the demands of justice. In so doing it should become clear why the distinction between facts and values, or between political science and political philosophy, is only useful up to a point.

Causes of ill-health and the health promotion agenda

As we have already seen, the causes of health, even if this term is understood narrowly, are broad ranging and include genetic, lifestyle, social and environmental components. These different factors, in combination, are used to explain types or instances of diseases like the cancers or heart diseases. In some cases the causal links are quite well understood and it is fairly easy to separate out the role of the different explanatory components, the classic instance being the causal link between the lifestyle factor of smoking and lung cancer. More frequently, for example with breast cancer, the chains of causation are not clear and it is difficult to separate the relative importance of the different kinds of explanatory factors. At one level this merely demonstrates the need for more epidemiology and other forms of medical research to try to trace causal chains. This is a matter of 'science', of developing better models and theories and testing them. But it is not as simple as that. The different kinds of explanation also have social and political dimensions.

If in the course of everyday conversation we were to hear that a friend had a disease which was genetic we might have a very different reaction from being told that it was a result of their personal lifestyle, or that it was caused by their working environment. In the first instance we would be inclined to see the disease as an unfortunate but naturally occurring imposition. In the case of it being work related we would be inclined to see the disease as a result of human action or neglect, and it would be almost instinctive to ask 'who is responsible?' even 'who is to blame?'. This illustrates the way in which explanation and politics are related.

Individuals attempting to get compensation for suffering diseases which they believe are related to their working environment immediately find themselves in the middle of disputes. Some of these may be about conflicting scientific evidence and theories, but some of them are between trade unions and employers, or between environmental groups and public authorities; and status, money and power play a significant part in these disputes. Because disease and ill-health does not occur alongside, and are somehow insulated from, other aspects of life, it cannot be understood in isolation from them. Institutions and policies are implicated in the causation and the management of ill-health, and therefore so are the politics of these institutions and policies.

Thus a large part of the debate about inequalities in health is about the social and political implications of the alternative explanations for inequalities. There are two main areas of debate. First, how far are the variations in health between social groups due to the different circumstances in which people live and work or to the different lifestyles that they adopt? Do people in deprived inner cities or other poor areas become ill because of pollution, damp housing, industrial accidents, and poverty, or because they smoke or drink more and eat an unhealthy diet? Second, even if some variations in health are due to behavioural factors, how far is this the result of choices that individuals make or how far are unhealthy lifestyles forced on people by their material and cultural environment?

A great deal of debate about models of health education and health promotion is really about alternative answers to these questions. Although many people will offer clear, and strongly felt, answers to these questions, they are in fact extremely difficult questions. They depend on becoming clear about the ideas of causality and responsibility, the relationships between them, and other complex philosophical issues.

The connection between the debate on causality and the debate about models of health promotion should be clear. They both rest on forming a view about who, if anyone, is responsible for ill-health. Who is responsible for bringing it about, and who is responsible for preventing or reducing it? Note that it is possible to distinguish between causal responsibility and moral responsibility for ill-health (Dworkin, 1981). Even in the case where a person is (partly) causally responsible, e.g. because of eating a certain diet, it does not automatically follow that they are morally responsible. That would be making a different sort of claim.

Obviously there is no straightforward answer to the questions above. We may give a different answer to the second than to the first, and we may vary our answer from case to case. It is likely that any sensible answer will spread responsibility out rather than assigning it all to one source, and some people may refuse to assign any responsibility at all. Despite these complexities the broad answer we give to these questions will shape the agenda of health promotion.

The key point is that it is impossible to decide on the agenda of health promotion in a purely technical way. There is no neutral method by which to decide what the objectives, processes or priorities should be, either in general or in specific cases. As we have seen, even identifying the causes of ill health depends on making political and philosophical judgements. The same applies to decisions about the most appropriate level and types of intervention (or more exactly combinations of intervention). How far is it fair or effective to encourage or expect individuals to change, rather than to aim for wide social changes?

The answer to this depends on *how* we work with the individual, but also on wider social and political issues. Sometimes people talk about assigning responsibility to individuals as 'victim blaming' and thereby condemn it. Yet it is equally common to hear about the importance of self empowerment, of helping individuals to make and take responsibility for their own decisions, including health-related ones. Superficially, these two approaches are at odds with each other, but it may be that on closer inspection they can be seen as complementary rather than conflicting, as throwing light on both the limitations and the importance of working with individuals. These complexities illustrate the importance of not relying on received ideas or slogans if we want to take a serious interest in health promotion issues.

Another dimension of the relationship between politics and health is the way in which political factors enter into the very conception of what counts as health or ill-health, or at least what is recognized as such by health services. Once again this can be approached through the idea of inequalities in health. All the reports into inequalities chart the fact that there are advantaged and disadvantaged with regard to access to health services. Class, race, and gender structure people's opportunities to benefit from health systems. Some of the reasons for this are clear; for example, having the freedom and the resources to negotiate and travel to appointments is a determinant of access. More generally, there is the fact that the range of services offered do not meet the range of needs of all groups in the population. Another aspect of this is language and language barriers to access. Those people who plan and deliver health care do not 'speak the same language' as everyone in the community. This can be taken both literally and metaphorically. In the literal sense the block on access is obvious, yet these blocks are just as real if we interpret language in the wider sense.

Systems of health care necessarily have values built into them. Some of these values relate to such fundamentals as what counts as a problem, and what are appropriate and acceptable ways of talking or behaving in order to get the best from the system. This need not imply conscious bias or discrimination on the part of health workers. But it does mean that there is an institutional and normative ethos that acts as a filter for demands and needs, in such a way that some people are effectively disadvantaged.

Justice and health promotion

If someone is in the 'health business' and it is clear to them that there is not enough health around, it is very tempting for them to come to firm conclusions about what needs to be done, and to carry it out sometimes without thinking through all of the implications of precisely what they are advocating. It is tempting to decide that everything should be organized so as to bring about the maximum amount of health.

We want to consider some of the objections to this line of thought, but before we do it is worth pointing out how intimately it connects with the idea of health promotion. Those who argue for healthy public policies are indeed saying that all policy – whether it relates to employment, taxation, transport, environment or whatever else – also relates to health and can and should be evaluated in terms of its consequences for health. The same can be said for the work of all sectors of society, and for the practices of individuals and communities both lay and professional. The use of health promotion as an umbrella term is meant to remind us of this. It works by giving us a new lens through which to view society (see Chapter 2).

But it is one thing to say that everything can be evaluated in terms of its contribution to health gain, and quite another to argue that everything should be organized so as to maximize health.

First, there is the problem of deciding what maximizing health means, partly because of the notoriously tricky question of the meaning of health as discussed in Chapter 1, and also because of the question of what is meant by 'maximizing'. These are by no means pedantic or merely academic concerns. Now that the language of health economics and of efficiency has become such a prominent part of the health land-scape, we are all affected by the ways in which these terms are inter-preted. Even if it were possible to produce some definitive measures of health which could be added together into totals (and let us stress the extraordinary conceptual and practical difficulties in this), there would still be uncertainty about the idea of maximization. Ought we to aim at maximizing the overall total, or the number of people above some target level, or the average level of health? Each of these would have different implications for policy and practice. Rival conceptions of the good society lie behind these alternatives. How far do we want to live in a society in which the high fliers can fly as high as humanly possible, or how far do we believe that substantial discrepancies in welfare are unfair or even undermine the quality of life for everyone? Here again we can see that it is impossible to by-pass our moral and political values.

This, however, is a problem of interpretation rather than an objection. The second problem amounts to a considerable objection, and can be summarized as follows: it is wrong to aim to maximize health because health is only one value among others. Health, in other words, does not deserve an automatic priority over other facets of life. It might be argued that those people who are pre-occupied with inequalities in health, and who wish to pursue greater social justice, are in danger of committing or causing other injustices. One of the weaknesses of the very broad con-ceptions of health – those conceptions in which health is equated with overall well-being – is that if we see all good things as components of health then it is not possible to have too much health, but in doing so we are obscuring basic questions about which combinations of these com-ponents are better or worse.

These basic questions are the stuff of social and political philosophy. There are many things that people value in addition to physical health. People are interested in and committed to relationships and careers, religious and artistic ends, personal projects and adventures, even when these things conflict with their health. It is true that a certain level of

good health is necessary to pursue many of these, but above this level it
is not true to say that extra health is valued more than other things.
Those people who ask for a short but happy life are expressing a perfectly intelligible desire, and one that we all identify with to some extent.
If individuals do not always give the pursuit of health absolute priority
then it is far from obvious that the state or health professionals should do
so on their behalf. Expenditure on schools, museums, galleries, leisure
centres, open spaces, transport systems and so on are all necessary for a
good life. Some of this expenditure will also contribute to health, but it is
a mistake to suppose that this is the sole criterion by which it should be
judged.

There is a similar problem with those activities that are damaging to
health. When should individuals or organizations be either encouraged
to, or made to, curtail such activities? Is it better for the state to regulate
the sale or consumption of foods and drugs for the sake of health and
safety, even if this entails restrictions on certain freedoms? If so what
should the boundaries of this kind of regulation be? Ought schoolchildren to be given a national diet as well as a national curriculum, and
if not why not? Sometimes this issue is highlighted by a particularly
dramatic or controversial case in which the pursuit of health comes into
conflict with respect for personal liberty, and often those with an
interest in health promotion would be the first to object. For example,
most people in health promotion would question the need and the
underlying motivation of the following:

> 'Once a person is HIV positive, we must make it unlawful for them to
> have sexual intercourse with anyone other than another HIV positive
> person. Disclosure must be mandatory. Anyone who breaches the
> rules would have to be quarantined.'

(Amiel, 1992)

It is just as important to be sceptical about more routine, and pro-
fessionally approved, health promotion interventions. However pure the
motive, it is easy to be blinkered by a focus on health.

By now it should have become clear that the family of values linked
with 'doing things in a health promoting way' (see Chapter 2) are not
always in constant harmony. The values of 'health', 'equality' and
'autonomy' are all strongly associated with health promotion. But more
of one does not always generate more of another. In particular, the
pursuit of health has to be qualified by a concern for equality, and by a
sometimes conflicting concern for autonomy.

Now it is also possible to return to the relationship between the mathematical and normative senses of 'inequality'. At the beginning of this chapter we raised the question of whether it is reasonable to merge the two senses and say that all variations in health are bad or morally unacceptable. In the light of the above discussion this is clearly controversial. At exactly what point patterns of mathematical 'inequality' in health are seen as unfair or unjust will depend on our value framework, on our vision of a good society and of the relative importance of health within it.

Power and health promotion

It is sometimes said that health workers, along with athletes and others, should stay out of politics. The fact that there are different conceptions of justice, and so different conceptions of the agenda and limits of health promotion, makes the call for neutrality highly problematic. However, debates about justice are not the only way in which social and political factors affect health promotion. Policies and practices are not only based on rational debate about what is good or fair (some would say they are not based on this at all!), but also on the ways in which these debates are structured and contained by power relations. What gets done is not necessarily what is judged best but what serves the interests of the most powerful.

This arises at both the macro and the micro-political levels referred to earlier. At the macro level there is the question of the role of the state, and the extent to which it can and should be independent from, and act as a corrective to, powerful forces in the wider society. There are all the questions about the formation of policies, and in what ways competing goals and interests are, consciously or unconsciously, represented and embodied in policies.

Equivalent questions arise at the micro level. Indeed, because particular settings are part of the wider world, the questions overlap and merge into one another in many respects. For example, a nurse practitioner working in health promotion clinics has to be aware of how the primary health care team might be using their relatively powerful position to try and impose their own health values on clients. But she also needs to be sensitive to the possibility that the team itself is being used as an instrument of government policy by, for example, being 'manipulated' by systems of funding.

The central point is that no policy (of government, institution, or professional group) is merely a neutral embodiment of good practice. All policies are expressions of values, and they are all shaped by processes in which some people have more power than others, and they have implications which (deliberately or otherwise) favour some people more than others.

To gain some insight into the concept of power it is worth reflecting on any setting (e.g. at home or at work) with which you are familiar. Let us, following the work of W.E. Connolly, say that one person (or group) has power over another person (or group) when the former limits the latter's autonomy. As we reflect on the ways in which this happens we see that the exercise of power does not necessarily entail the deliberate or overt use of force.

Connolly (1974) identifies six forms of power: use of force, coercion, manipulation, deterrence, anticipatory surrender and conditioning. These differ in the degree to which they are overt, active or deliberate, and whether they limit actions or thoughts. You can make someone do something, you can put pressure on someone, you can trick them, you can establish a hostile or threatening climate knowingly or unknowingly, or certain courses of action can be literally unthinkable. Thus power is not only about stopping or making people do things, it is about limiting what is discussed, how things are discussed, and even what people know and how they think. It has a visible and an invisible aspect. We can apply this to the power relationships within and between groups of health workers.

Take the idea of a health care team in which decisions are supposed to be made through open discussion. What are the subtle and the less subtle ways in which power can be manifest in this process? A common consequence of professional power relations is that individual workers feel an inner conflict between their own personal beliefs and values and those which dominate their work setting. Indeed, it is quite possible for the majority of workers in a particular setting to feel unhappy with the philosophy underlying their practice. This fact alone illustrates the constraints that can be exercised by the power of others or by systems of management and funding. Once we have some insight into this we can begin to imagine the situation of the patient or client who typically has little or no power, is in an unfamiliar world, is anxious, and may be unwell. In this situation the potential for limiting autonomy and imposing values is huge, and all the more so when this can be done in the name of health promotion.

Thus the idea that a health worker should stay out of politics is absurd. Of course there are serious doubts about whether it is appropriate for someone to use their work as an opportunity for propaganda. But simply by doing their job all health workers are inevitably in the midst of a network of political processes. Power is being exercised over them and through them. The only options are to choose ignorance or to try to develop political understanding and skills.

References

Amiel, B. (1992) AIDS flourishes in a culture of soft soap. *The Sunday Times,* 9 June.

Connolly, W.E. (1974) *The Terms of Political Discourse.* Heath, Lexington, Mass.

Dworkin, G. (1981) Voluntary Health Risks and Public Policy. *The Hastings Center Report,* 11 (5).

French, J. (1990) Boundaries and Horizons, the role of health education within health promotion. *Health Education Journal* **49** (1).

Smith, G.D., Bartley, M., & Blane, D. (1990) The Black Report on socioeconomic inequalities in health ten years on. *British Medical Journal,* 301, 373–7.

Townsend, P., Davidson, N., & Whitehead, M. (1988) *Inequalities in Health: The Black Report/The Health Divide,* Penguin Books, Harmondsworth.

Further reading

Research Unit in Health and Behavioural Change, University of Edinburgh (1989) *Changing the public health* John Wiley and Sons Ltd, Chichester.

Rodmell, S. & Watt, A. (Eds) (1986) *The Politics of Health Education. Raising the Issues.* Routledge and Kegan Paul, London.

Townsend, P., Davidson, N. & Whitehead, M. (1988) *Inequalities in Health: The Black Report/The Health Divide,* Penguin Books.

Chapter 4
Ethical Issues in Health Promotion

Most nurses are familiar with the ethical dilemmas commonly confronted in practice. Issues such as euthanasia, abortion and informed consent to research, readily spring to mind. Of less salience, but no less challenging, are the ethical issues raised by health promotion. Questions such as: 'Who should be informed about a person's HIV status?'; 'Should we fluoridate all water supplies?'; 'What should be done about a GP who frequently drinks to excess?'; and 'Should nurses be involved in political action to reduce unemployment because of its detrimental effect on health?' These questions demonstrate the importance of such debate.

Discussion of these issues has not been extensive when compared to the attention paid to the more traditional ethical concerns. This chapter helps to rectify this in a small way by exploring some of the ethical issues in health promotion work by nurses. The first part of the chapter considers examples of health promotion from the four branches of nursing: adult nursing, nursing those with learning disabilities, mental health nursing and nursing with children. The examples link quite closely with later chapters in the book which look at these areas, thus enabling us to explore not only practice but the ethical implications. The second part of the chapter builds on these examples and puts forward a number of questions which may help us as we think about the ethical dimensions of any health promotion work that we may be engaged in.

Health promotion with adults: helping people to stop smoking

Scenario

A sister working on a cardiac unit came across a research paper by Rowe & Macleod Clark (1993) which discusses how nurses might assist patients in giving up smoking. She decided to consider implementing a similar programme in the unit. A meeting with nursing staff was arranged to discuss the idea and as a result a number of issues were raised.

The sister began the meeting by explaining how each member of the nursing team would be given the opportunity to go on a course to learn more about the programme and how it worked in practice. A second year student nurse expressed relief at this as all her attempts at advising people to stop smoking or to try and cut down had so far failed. The final year student nurse was concerned that patients should not be forced to give up smoking.

The sister explained that the research study had only included patients who very much wanted to stop smoking; the remainder of patients would not participate in the programme. The student confessed that she still had some qualms about the idea because some of the patients might feel pressurized to join in even if they did not really want to.

The staff nurse on the unit said she was reluctant to participate in the programme for two reasons. She was a smoker herself and had tried, unsuccessfully, on several occasions to give up. She said she would feel a fraud trying to help patients to give up. Her other reservation was that the patients themselves might end up feeling even more guilty than they already did. Patients who did not feel they wanted to give up smoking or could give up, would feel bad, and any patient who failed on the programme would feel even worse.

At this point the senior staff nurse, who had so far not said anything, suggested that some of the patients not involved in the programme might feel neglected. She also asked whether the programme would mean that the patients' smoking room would be converted to a non-smoking area? The senior staff nurse then admitted that she felt she was fighting a losing battle against smoking with all the advertising everywhere and the government's refusal to ban it.

The sister drew the meeting to a close and it was decided that each member of the team would read Rowe & Macleod Clark's paper and give the matter some further thought. They arranged to meet again in a week.

Let us now examine some of the ethical issues raised by this scenario. A key issue here is the one mentioned by the final year student nurse about *whether patients should be forced to give up smoking*. Rowe & Macleod Clark's programme does not coerce people in this way as patients are invited to be part of the scheme on the basis of their expressed desire to quit smoking. A more subtle form of coercion might, however, operate even with this scheme: for example, if patients feel unduly pressurized to participate because of the manner in which they are invited to join. In addition, covert coercion might occur because patients feel intimidated by the health care setting more generally and are encouraged to comply so as to please health care staff. Alternatively, pressure may exist because they feel some anxiety about jeopardizing their future care if they do not seem to be co-operating with their 'treatment'. An extreme example of the latter would be the case of a

consultant surgeon who refuses to operate on his patients unless they
quit smoking prior to surgery.

Closely linked to this question of the degree of coercion involved in
the programme is the need to respect people's autonomy. This might
include their *right to choose to smoke*, even if this is health damaging.
The question of whether the patient's smoking room would be converted
to a non-smoking area is relevant here. If it is, and there is not a convenient substitute for those wishing to smoke, this might be interpreted
as an infringement of the smoking patients' liberty, or in contrast as a
legitimate act of paternalism designed to protect the smokers' health. If
the door of the smoking room was frequently left open and the smoke
polluted neighbouring beds, then the question is raised of whether it is
possible to restrict the freedom of one individual to avoid damaging the
health prospects of another. In this case, should a person who smokes be
restricted, to avoid harming another through passive smoking? The same
issue would occur if there was only one patients' day room in the unit
where smokers and non-smokers alike shared facilities. The tension in
this instance is between personal freedom and the common good.

The balance between *doing good and not causing harm*, or beneficence and non-maleficence, is another ethical issue raised by the scenario. The staff nurse is referring to this when she suggests that patients
who do not join the programme might feel even more guilty than they
already do, and those who join the programme but do not succeed in
quitting smoking may also suffer in some respect. The ethical issue here
is how can we weigh the possible benefits of the programme against the
possible harms?

The need for adequate training for new initiatives like this one is also
linked to beneficence and non-maleficence. In the scenario, it seems the
nurses will be prepared for this role through the course mentioned by
the sister. The importance of this is highlighted by the student nurse who
acknowledges her history of failure to help patients to either cut down or
quit smoking. Inadequate or non-existent training for a role may mean
that practitioners cause more harm than good in their attempts to help.
The fact that the programme is based on empirical research rather than
custom and practice may also contribute to our ethical evaluation that it
is 'a good thing'. But empirical research is only valuable if it, also, considers the full range of benefits and harms.

The senior staff nurse also expressed concern about the patients who
did not join the stop smoking programme, arguing that they might feel
neglected. The concern here is the *fair* or just distribution of health care
resources, in this case nursing expertise and time. Which is the most
equitable response in this instance: to spend more time with the patients
who feel they would like to stop smoking in an attempt to improve their

health, or to focus on the remaining smokers, who might be considered in greater need?

The senior staff nurse's other frustration regarding tobacco advertising raises the interesting dilemma about the balance of responsibility between action to improve health at the *individual level or the societal level*? When there is evidence that a ban on tobacco advertising might have a beneficial effect on the uptake and continuance of smoking, is it ethically acceptable to focus primarily on individual change? What is the responsibility of a government in promoting the health of its citizens? What should be done when measures to enhance the physical health of one group, i.e. people who smoke, conflict with measures which contribute to the mental and social health of another group, i.e. those who work in the tobacco industry?

The final ethical issue to be discussed in this context concerns the question of role models. The staff nurse who is herself a smoker does not wish to be involved in the programme. *Is it ethically acceptable for a nurse who smokes to be involved in a stop smoking programme*? Some might see the nurse who smokes as neglecting her responsibility to act as a role model in health promotion, or as acting deceptively if she does not inform the patients that she herself is a smoker. If she does inform the patients, the effectiveness of the programme might be enhanced as patients identify with someone who fully understands the difficulties of giving up smoking. Alternatively, the effectiveness of the programme might be reduced as she lacks credibility in this particular role. Her presence on the programme might be viewed as undermining the commitment of the unit to no-smoking. Alternatively it may be interpreted as visible proof of the unit's respect for a person's right to smoke, thereby possibly benefiting patients not participating in the programme.

Health promotion with people with learning disabilities: working towards an ordinary life

Scenario

For her thirty-ninth birthday Teresa had a new teddy bear. She was delighted with it, eagerly showing it to the woman who came to read the electricity meter. The community nurse (learning disabilities) was also told all about the bear when she visited Teresa and her elderly mother. The nurse was compiling a register of people with learning disabilities and was interested to find out more about Teresa's life with her mother.

Mrs O'Leary was now in her late seventies but still enjoyed good health. She looked after Teresa alone and had done so for over ten years since her husband died suddenly with a heart attack. Mrs O'Leary was proud of the way she had adapted to Teresa's unexpected arrival all those years ago and had done her best to cope when she realized that her daughter would 'never grow up', as she put it. Teresa attended a day centre on two mornings a week, where she had learned to cook and had acquired other new skills like using a telephone. The community nurse was keen to extend Teresa's experience and was aware of a new group starting in the area. She told Mrs O'Leary and Teresa about the group and when both seemed interested, invited Teresa to go along. Mrs O'Leary seemed slightly concerned about the change in Teresa's routine, but ever mindful of the question 'what will happen when I'm gone?' she agreed to let Teresa go. Teresa herself was initially worried about the new group but soon became very enthusiastic about it.

One evening Teresa returned full of delight, but Mrs O'Leary was horrified to see that she was wearing make-up. A beauty therapist had visited the group and the women had been shown how to make themselves up. Teresa had volunteered to be the model. [The particular difficulty of teaching women with learning difficulties to use make-up was identified by Walsh (1988) and discussed by Voysey (1993).] Mrs O'Leary immediately picked up the phone and rang the community nurse to express her unhappiness at what had happened; she was sure there must be some mistake. The community nurse tried to pacify Mrs O'Leary, explaining how the whole group aimed to build up participants' esteem and that despite the fact that Teresa was still very much a child in some ways, in others she was a thirty-nine year old woman and at times needed to be allowed to behave as such. Mrs O'Leary was outraged at this suggestion and told the nurse that, as her mother, she knew what was best for Teresa. In tears, as she put the phone down, she shouted, 'You'll be suggesting she have a boyfriend or be sterilized next!'

Let us examine some of the ethical issues raised by this scenario. A key dilemma here is, *who should decide what is in Teresa's best interests*? Is it Teresa herself, Mrs O'Leary or the community nurse? The current ethos in caring for people with learning disabilities is that people like Teresa should as far as possible be enabled to lead an ordinary life. They should therefore be allowed, among other things, the *right to choose* and make decisions about things which affect them. It seems from the scenario that Teresa did choose to wear make-up when given the opportunity.

The difficult question becomes, is she capable of exercising choice and coping with the consequences of choice, in this and other areas of her life? If she expresses a desire to develop a relationship with a man, is she in a position to make that choice? If she wants to develop a sexual relationship should she have that right? Some people would suggest that the degree of *informed choice* taking place is a significant indicator of Teresa's autonomy in this situation. In other words, is Teresa capable of understanding the consequences of intimate personal relationships or of a sexual encounter? If she is, then she may choose and be helped to cope with the consequences of her choice; if she is not, then others should act on her behalf.

Other people would see this restriction on the free choice of people with learning disabilities as perpetuating society's discriminatory attitudes, suggesting that in order to earn, for example, the privilege of being a parent, one must possess certain 'qualifications.' This they feel smacks somewhat of eugenics with its quest for a perfect race and all its unpleasant connotations.

The community nurse feels that previously people with learning disabilities have suffered great inequalities, which it is time now for society to rectify. Her work is therefore a small contribution to *justice*. The nurse sees this work being best achieved by enabling Teresa to participate in her care, thereby demonstrating *respect for Teresa as a person*. Her assessment of Teresa's situation was that she might benefit from the widened experience of attending the new local group in addition to the day centre; once again the moral principle of *beneficence* appears. A difficulty of respecting Teresa as a person is that it involves taking risks in a way that would previously have been unheard of. Thus if Mrs O'Leary's fears come to fruition, Teresa might risk pregnancy or some form of sexual abuse or exploitation. Another perhaps less significant but potentially more pervasive form of harm engendered by this approach, might be that people like Teresa have their expectations inappropriately raised when there is no realistic opportunity for fulfilment.

Mrs O'Leary's perspective is different from that of the community nurse. Her concern is to *protect Teresa from harm* so she acts *paternalistically* on behalf of Teresa, in what she as her mother feels are Teresa's best interests. Some might criticize Mrs O'Leary as having an 'eternal child' image of Teresa, petrifying her as an asexual being. Others might support Mrs O'Leary as exercizing her right as a parent to decide what is in her child's best interest, free from outside interference. She has successfully looked after Teresa on her own all these years; what right do 'professionals' now have to come and 'upset things'?

Implicit within the differing perceptions of the community nurse and Mrs O'Leary are contrasting ideas about what it means to promote Teresa's well-being. The question here becomes: *Is autonomy (and how much autonomy) an integral part of human health and well-being?* Mrs O'Leary feels that Teresa's well-being will be best promoted in a place of refuge and safety in the world, because of her learning difficulties. In other words she needs an asylum where her vulnerability may not be exploited and where she can enjoy life to the full within her limitations.

The community nurse sees the way to promote Teresa's well-being in very different terms. Teresa does have a learning disability but this should not mean that this limits *every* area of her life. As far as possible, Teresa's autonomy should be respected; she should be allowed to participate in decision-making in everything from how she is employed, who her friends are and whether she has a partner, to how she spends her spare time, what education she receives and where she lives. The ethical dilemma is which conception of well-being ought we to be working towards?

The final ethical concern to arise from this scenario concerns *the degree of participation* in the endeavour. It can be suggested that the nurse's attempts to encourage Teresa and her mother to participate in the decision about attending the new group were a failure. It seems Mrs O'Leary was unaware of the purpose of the group and its programme. Was the nurse behaving in an ethical fashion given this lack of *informed* consent? The same question arises more generally when we consider how this new 'ordinary life' philosophy in the care of people with learning difficulties came to be adopted as 'a good thing'? Was it through a democratic process or did an elite group, possibly of professionals, impose it on a sometimes unwilling group of vulnerable people and their carers? It seems from the scenario that Teresa is partially persuaded of its worth; Mrs O'Leary, however, is not. Given the possible lack of *democratic* participation here, does this make the 'ordinary life' philosophy unethical?

Mental health promotion: early detection of depression in primary care

Scenario

Six months ago Nigel was made redundant from his job as a driver for a bakery. Since then he has applied for many jobs but with no success, the majority of his applications not even receiving an acknowledgement. Nigel is asthmatic and regularly visits his local surgery where a health promotion clinic for asthma sufferers is run by the GP and the practice nurse. The surgery, like all the neighbourhood, reeks of decay. When he was driving, Nigel used not to notice the drabness of his inner city surroundings. More recently they seem increasingly grey to him, threatening to almost suffocate him on his worst days.

Although she works in a single-handed practice, the practice nurse is keen to try and offer the best care she can to the patients. Recently she has introduced the use of mood questionnaires – for the early detection of depression –

at all the health promotion clinics running at the surgery. By asking patients about their sleep pattern, level of anxiety and how they are feeling, she hopes to be able to identify people suffering with depression who otherwise might have been missed. The practice nurse is aware of Nigel's redundancy and has always been impressed by his positive outlook. She was therefore surprised to discover, when using the mood questionnaire with him that he might actually be depressed.

She asked Nigel to wait in the clinic while she discussed this with the GP. The GP decided to deal with the matter straight away and spoke to Nigel, suggesting he might like to try an anti-depressant, Fluoxetine. Nigel was quite taken aback at the GP's suggestion. He had not really seen himself as being depressed and in need of any tablets; he was much more concerned to keep on top of his asthma and get a job. In the hurry of the clinic, however, there was not much opportunity for Nigel to discuss his views. The GP quickly wrote a prescription and as he handed it to Nigel he mentioned that Nigel should not drive while taking the medication and he was to make an appointment for two weeks' time to see him again.

Nigel took the Fluoxetine but soon found himself feeling nauseated, with bad headaches. The more he reflected on the idea of being thought of as depressed, the less he liked it. He was particularly fed up that taking Fluoxetine meant he was unable to drive. How could he possibly get another job if he could not drive? He was also concerned that mention of two health problems on any application form – asthma *and* depression – would mean he would not even be given a chance to prove himself with a new employer. Nigel never made his two week follow-up appointment. He threw the rest of the tablets down the toilet. 'I am going to cope with this my own way', he thought.

Let us consider the ethical issues raised by this scenario. Perhaps the most striking feature of this account is the way in which Nigel sought help for one health problem and in so doing unwittingly allowed himself to be diagnosed as having quite a different additional problem. It might be possible to see the use of the mood questionnaire by the practice nurse as an invasion of Nigel's *privacy*. The ethical question here is how far can we *intervene in peoples' lives* for the sake of health promotion? We might wish to see Nigel giving his *informed consent* to the questionnaire prior to its use, or we might see his registration with a GP as implicit consent to participation in all health care activities. We do not hesitate to resuscitate a victim of a car accident simply because we have not asked their permission; why should diagnosis of depression be any different? Alternatively, we might argue that the accident victim's life is in danger, whereas at the moment Nigel's is not.

Linked to these issues is the question of whether Nigel was in fact being *coerced* by what happened at the clinic. Certainly it appears he did not *freely choose* to have his mental health assessed in this way; he was unaware of the implications of what was happening. The manner in which his medication was prescribed allowed for little *participation* and may therefore have failed to *respect his autonomy*.

It can of course be suggested, in contrast to the above interpretation, that the GP and practice nurse were acting in Nigel's best interest. They were motivated by duties of *beneficence*. Early detection of depression does seem to mean that recovery is hastened and the possible future harms, of suicide and inability to work through severe depression, avoided. These ideas are explored in Chapter 7. Supporters of this view might also ask: would it be acceptable, now we have tools like these, to fail to use them simply because patients have not given permission? Are we not duty bound to make use of the best available for patients? Indeed, is it feasible to gain all patients' permission?

Balanced against these potential benefits from the early detection of depression are possible *harms from the intervention*. Labelling some-one as depressed, in need of medication and mentally ill in some sense, admits them to a very stigmatized status in our society. This was Nigel's concern when he thought having 'depression' on his job application might deter potential employers. Indeed the stigma of mental illness might also be linked to his own reluctance to label himself in this way, denial and concealment being seen by him as less socially 'costly' approaches. Other possible harms are linked to side effects of medi-cation which, as Nigel found, are at their worst in the first few weeks, and the limitation placed on his life and livelihood by not being allowed to drive.

In the scenario, it seems the value placed on health by the pro-fessionals and by Nigel himself are at odds. The practice nurse and the GP assume unthinkingly that elimination of depression will be salient in Nigel's life. In contrast, Nigel balances this against his desire for a job. The professionals might be accused of *healthism* here, i.e. believing health to be the supreme goal which must override all other aims human beings might pursue.

In any case Nigel might feel that his approach is much more health promoting because if he secures a job, his depression, which appears to be related to his unemployment, might abate. In some ways being unable to drive and placing oneself in a stigmatized category might prove very health diminishing in this particular situation. Closely linked to this is the question of whether it is ethically acceptable to ignore the *broader societal issues* in this scenario. By not focusing on unemployment as something to be tackled by health promoters, but on depression in the individual that is a consequence of unemployment, the health worker may be guilty of both victim blaming and using inappropriate methods of work.

Promoting children's health: learning about healthy eating

Scenario

Mrs Dukes had thought about nursing as a career before going into teaching. Even now she still had an interest in health and strongly believed in the health education work that a school might do. In her five years at the junior school Mrs Dukes had got to know the school nurse, Clare Smart, quite well. They had occasionally talked about the idea of working together with the children on a health education project; maybe now the time had come.

When Clare was at the school to carry out some routine vision tests Mrs Dukes raised the subject again. Clare mentioned that the Health Authority's Health Promotion Unit was just launching a healthy eating campaign and she wondered if the school project should tie in with that. It was not long before they were enthusiastically planning a morning's session with the children. All 20 children would be asked to bring in an item of healthy and unhealthy food. They planned to base some games and exercises about a healthy diet around these items. By the end of the morning they hoped all the children would have some understanding about the importance of eating a high fibre, low fat, salt and sugar diet.

On the morning of the project the classroom was full of all kinds of food from tins of baked beans and packets of crisps, to apples and chocolate bars. The children were highly excited; they loved it when they had to bring in something from home. Only one boy, Paul, came with nothing; he said his Mum had not had time to get him anything. Mrs Dukes gave him a potato and a can of fizzy drink. She knew Paul's family were finding it difficult to make ends meet since his Dad had become ill, and she did not want Paul to feel the odd one out.

The day began with the children putting all their unhealthy food on a table covered with black paper and their healthy food on another table covered with white paper. They then looked at both piles and led by Mrs Dukes and Clare discussed why each item was either healthy or unhealthy. Chocolate, fizzy drinks and crisps were immediately awarded an unhealthy label. Apples, wholemeal bread and fresh orange juice were unanimously agreed to be healthy.

Arguments arose, however, when a can of diet lemonade was found on the healthy table. Lucy, who had brought the can, said her Mum said it was healthy because it was diet lemonade and did not have sugar. Peter, who said his Mum was a dietician, said it had artificial sweeteners in it that were unhealthy. A louder dispute arose when the sunflower margarine was found alongside some butter on the healthy table. Peter had brought the sunflower margarine but Imogen had donated the butter. Peter said the butter had the wrong sort of fat in it and was unhealthy. Imogen said her Mum knew a lot about diets and she said butter was healthy. Her Mum had read in a magazine that there is no such thing as the wrong type of fat; they are all good for you.

At this point Mrs Dukes decided it was time for a break; neither she nor Clare Smart had expected it to be such a noisy and argumentative session.

Let us explore some of the ethical issues raised by this healthy eating project. A central question surrounds the degree of certainty about what actually constitutes a healthy diet. In the scenario, artificial sweeteners and fat appear to be areas of considerable controversy. The ethical question is, should we be educating children in this way if there is some *uncertainty about the factual basis* of what is being taught? In support of continued education, for example about fat, there is the view that we do have some evidence that a diet high in saturated fat may predispose to heart disease. Given the importance of early eating patterns and the significance of heart disease as a health problem, we are morally obliged to act on this knowledge so that people might thereby *benefit*.

In contrast to this is the view that the aetiology of heart disease is complex; there are some indications that saturated fat may be implicated but the evidence is conflicting. Until we have a clearer picture of what is happening we should not educate people to alter their diet as this may turn out to be misinformation and therefore *harmful*.

It would be interesting to know more of how Mrs Dukes and Clare Smart dealt with these classroom conflicts. If they used them as an opportunity to explore the controversies surrounding a healthy diet, then we might see this as being *honest* with the children. Alternatively, we might see exposure to these uncertainties with all their complexities as capable of *harming* the children by creating confusion.

A second ethical issue concerns the extent to which the children are *able to act* on this new knowledge and alter their diet. A key issue here is that children are not wholly responsible for their diet. Parents obviously play a powerful mediating role. One can imagine cases where some parents would be very responsive to a child's concern to eat a healthy diet, assuming this to be the outcome of the session.

Alternatively, one can imagine those who are more reluctant for a variety of reasons. Some parents might feel strongly that suggestions from the school that the family diet be altered are intrusive and an *invasion of privacy*. In keeping with this, it might be argued that the parents did not *consent* to the healthy eating programme in an informed way. Others, however, might see the sending of foodstuffs to school as implicit consent to participate in a healthy eating campaign. Another family might be unable to afford a healthy diet or might lack the time for healthy food preparation. In this sense, the project may be accused of *victim blaming* where the children's *consciousness is raised* while failing to equip them with the means to alter their diet.

Paul was the child whose parents were unable to afford to give him anything to take into school for the project. Fortunately Mrs Dukes was sensitive enough to try and minimize his embarassment by giving him the potato and fizzy drink. Had this not been the case an ethical objection to this kind of project might be that they perpetuate disadvantage, with their dependence on parental resources. In this way the project could be seen as *unjust*. In another sense, by treating Paul the same as the other children in the class, by enabling him also to be aware of the constituents of a healthy diet despite his disadvantaged economic position, it might be possible to view the project as working towards a *fairer* world.

The last ethical issue raised by the scenario concerns the degree of coercion it involved. It seems that neither the children nor their parents were given a *free choice* about their participation in the healthy eating project. Some might see this concern as unnecessarily pedantic given that health education is an 'obvious good' and that children are obliged by law to participate in an educational process. (Compulsory education is therefore an example where the freedom of the individual is curtailed for what is perceived to be his or her own good – a paternalistic judgement by the state.) If we think of other more controversial examples within health education, like sex education, then the parent's but not really the child's right to free choice and consent is sometimes recognized. Should this need for consent be extended to other spheres of health promotion in the educational setting?

Each of these scenarios has raised ethical dilemmas. We have not attempted to resolve them here, but merely to set out the range of relevant issues and principles. It is worth reflecting on our own position in relation to these and other health promotion scenarios. To help us do this the remainder of the chapter will consider a number of questions which may be used as we think about the ethical dimensions of any health promotion work that we are engaged in.

Elements of ethical evaluation

The central ethical question for health promoters is the one which runs through the whole of this part of the book: 'What do we mean by health and well-being? What is our vision of a full life and a flourishing society?'

Below are some other questions which can be used as prompts to thought. The answers to them do not tell us in a straightforward way what is ethically acceptable or unacceptable. They cannot be used as a formula for ethical decision making, but they are designed to help us explore, and reflect on, the range of considerations that are relevant to ethically evaluating health promotion. Some of them will seem more relevant to some interventions than others, but most of them are relevant to most interventions. They are not intended to be exhaustive; as we think about them, and as we try to answer them in specific cases, other questions will come to mind.

We have said that these are questions to ask about 'interventions'. It is because health promotion involves intervening in the lives of people that it raises ethical questions. It can be argued that all activities, however private or small-scale, raise ethical questions, but it is plausible to argue that they do so only to the extent that they have implications for harming or benefiting humans or other forms of life. Health promotion interventions are deliberately undertaken in order to make a significant difference to the experiences and life chances of people. Health workers or others who initiate them should be able to give an account of why they are worthwhile, why they are acceptable, and what risks or potential harm accompany them. Being able to give such an account is the central part of what it means to be *accountable*.

While reading through these questions and the explanatory comments and examples, it might be worth relating them to one or two interventions with which you are familiar. By intervention we mean either a specific instance of practice, or a programme or a general policy. Each question gives us an important element of ethical thinking. It is important to recognize that our intuitions and judgements will vary considerably from case to case. This is because we are evaluating the *combination* of elements, and not each element separately.

How coercive is the intervention?

How far is the targeted individual or group forced to fit in with the objectives of the health promoter? As we have seen, this relationship is typically one in which there is an inequality in power. The agency responsible may be a health professional, or someone else in a position of relative authority such as a teacher, or may even be local or national government. In all these cases it is possible to imagine degrees of coerciveness in which the power relation is exercised more or less. At one extreme are interventions which are entirely voluntary, and at the other extreme interventions which are effectively compulsory. Some may doubt the possibility of completely avoiding pressure but close to this end of the spectrum would be certain kinds of educational interventions where both the objectives and methods are aimed at empowerment. At the other extreme would be health promotion imposed by law (e.g. food and drug legislation, seatbelt legislation).

This sort of pressure to comply, and the threat of sanctions, can also apply in health care settings where there are strictly imposed rules (e.g. no smoking). Most interventions are likely to fall somewhere in the middle. Coercion is too crude a word to convey all the different kinds of 'pressure' that might be brought to bear, and we may, for example, have different ethical intuitions about the use of 'incentives' rather than sanctions.

How overt is any coercion?

The idea of degrees of powerful pressure only captures some of our instincts about the ethics of persuasion or manipulation. One other dimension is the question of openness or transparency. Power is often hidden, and sometimes deliberately so, from the target of actions. There seems to be moral difference between openly, and with the full aware-ness of both parties, threatening or imposing a sanction, and more subtle and less self-conscious forms of manipulation, such as if health pro-fessionals take advantage of their greater confidence or knowledge of the facts to present a partial picture to clients in order to promote certain objectives. Even assuming that this is being done in the interests of the client's health (which we would take to be the normal case), it would amount to an exercise of power which needs some kind of justification. It may be a deliberate act of paternalism, or it may be that certain habits of thought or behaviour are built into institutions or policies.

Who is the intervention designed to benefit?

It might be assumed that the target and the intended beneficiary are always the same, but this is not so. One class of exceptions is where the target is other carers, such as relatives. Here demands might be made which do not directly benefit the target group, but benefit them indirectly insofar as they are assumed to have a stake in the welfare of others.

Another class of exceptions is when both the target individuals and a wider group of people stand to benefit. It is normally assumed that if someone is damaging or risking their own health we have less grounds for interfering than if they are harming the health of others. The main reason many people support restrictions on smoking in public places is the threat to health from passive smoking. However there are, pre-sumably, limits to how far we feel individuals are responsible for the welfare of others, and even narrower limits to how far they can be held responsible. Even when we are dealing with the 'soft' area of health education, we need to sort out who the education is designed to benefit. Are we educating people to look after themselves, or their families, or society at large? Or how much of each?

What is the cost-benefit ratio?

Interventions are aimed at producing benefit but they inevitably have a cost. The obvious cost is the economic price of the resources that have to be devoted to the intervention. Clearly if the benefit achieved is very small and the cost very high it makes sense to review the overall worth of the intervention. This is an ethical issue and not just an economic one, because the key question is: 'What other, more effective, ends might these resources be put to?'. This is the question of economic efficiency which some may feel has been too dominant in recent debates about health care values, but it is one important element of evaluation.

The question about costs and benefits must be interpreted more broadly. Interventions have a personal and social cost as well as an economic one. Even sitting down and talking with someone can give rise to feelings of guilt, regret or anxiety as well as any intended benefits. If we consider large scale interventions, like immunisation or screening programmes, then we can see a whole complex of costs and benefits. Many people may pay some small price for the benefit of others. It is no good judging policies or practices simply in terms of the good they do; we always have to consider the overall consequences, and must be prepared to ask whether the cost is too high.

What is the distribution of costs and benefits?

As we saw in Chapter 3 a key issue for all health workers is the extent to which they ought to be involved in working for a fairer society. Because health promotion is often proactive rather than reactive, it is possible for health promoters to build ends like equity into their targets. This sort of commitment can be more or less radical, ranging from trying to ensure equal access to health care institutions to trying to minimize inequalities in health itself.

Any of these positions rest upon (highly contestable) ethical standpoints. One way of bringing these issues into sharp focus is to ask about the justification, and the limits, of targeting the health promoter's time, effort or resources. How far is it acceptable for a manager or a practitioner working in a community (or health care setting) to concentrate their attention on the most disadvantaged?

There are two possible objections. First, any model of disadvantage or need is likely to be a blunt instrument and may result in equally serious need being overlooked. Second, individuals with other real (but perhaps less serious) needs may feel that they have an equal claim for attention. This is particularly likely to be true where people feel that they are paying for the service through tax and insurance. The issues here are very complicated because the values of equal access, equality in health and respect for demands tend to conflict. But this complexity makes it all the more necessary for health promoters to ask these questions about interventions, and at least to try to make their own positions explicit.

How secure is the knowledge base?

All interventions rest on two assumptions: that the immediate objective is a good thing, and that the methods being employed to attain these objectives will bring them about. For example, the promotion of condoms for the prevention of HIV transmission assumes that condoms are (to some degree) effective for this role, and that the measures that are taken to promote them will have some effect on their use.

As far as possible we aim to ensure that these assumptions are based on research evidence; in other words they rest on a knowledge base about health and health promotion. But it is notoriously the case that this knowledge base is subject to revision, and is much more secure in some places than in others. Different sorts of knowledge make up this base. The assumptions about health are likely to be based on the biological sciences, whereas the assumptions about interventions are always partly based on the social sciences where the evidence and the theoretical models tend to be controversial. However, controversy on both these is widespread. The controversy about the overall risks and benefits of the contraceptive pill, or of different diets, is an example of the first. The controversy about the merits of large scale short-term campaigns (e.g. national no smoking day) an example of the second.

It seems that an intervention based on a relatively insecure knowledge base is, other things being equal, more ethically dubious. The less confidence we have in doing good the greater the risk of doing harm overall.

Who decides to intervene, and how?

This is a question about the process of the decision rather than its content. Given that there is always a cost to interventions, and that there is room for controversy about the merits of health promotion practice, it is worth asking who is best placed to make decisions on them. In the health promotion literature the emphasis on participation is itself a sign that 'experts' or professionals are not always the best people to decide. In many areas of health care a great deal of weight is put on the ethical importance of informed choice. In these cases we judge that individuals who are most directly affected by the intervention (e.g. surgery) should at least have a veto on what is done 'for their sake'.

Things are not always so clear cut in other areas. For example, if a health worker feels that listening to and acknowledging the feelings of a client would be beneficial is he or she supposed to talk that proposed intervention through with the client? It is easy to imagine circumstances in which this could be counter-productive. Nonetheless it seems right that as far as possible interventions should not simply be imposed on the target group, but some form of consultation and negotiation should take place. It is often possible to do this directly when the proposed intervention is face-to-face, but some health promotion interventions are large scale and are designed to have an impact on people who cannot be consulted directly.

This is certainly the case with policy interventions such as banning forms of advertising, or taxing unhealthy products. Here the issue is about the political legitimacy of the decision, e.g. have democratic mechanisms been employed in the decision-making process? The same questions can be asked about the policy decisions of local or small-scale institutions.

Making ethical judgements

The above questions are only prompts to thought, and given an actual or possible intervention we could attempt to answer them. These answers will not dictate, but only suggest, an ethical evaluation, for a number of reasons.

First, all of these questions have a factual or empirical component. There is a great deal of scope for disagreement here, which does not arise from different ethical outlooks but entirely from different interpretations of the facts. Second, only some of the questions (e.g. the cost-benefit ratio, and the security of the knowledge base) have relatively clear-cut ethical implications, i.e. there would be a broad consensus about their role in evaluation (others things being equal, the lower the cost benefit ratio and the more secure the knowledge base, the better).

The answers to other questions (e.g. who the intervention is designed to benefit, and the security of the knowledge base) would not necessarily have the same ethical implications to everyone; it would depend on what underlying values or principles they gave priority to. If someone regards the pursuit of social justice as a very important, possibly even overriding, value, then they may be supportive of an intervention which redistributes resources across society. Other people may see the same intervention as an illegitimate violation of individuals' property and freedom.

Thus we can see that we cannot *derive* our ethical framework from answering these questions. Rather they are intended to help us to be explicit about the elements of our individual or collective frameworks, and to encourage critical reflection on these frameworks. If we want to justify our ethical judgements the first step is to be able to articulate the principles and values which are implicit in the practical judgements we make (and, if possible, the priority relations between these values).

Making these values and principles explicit is far from easy. It soon becomes apparent that behind mundane or routine actions lie whole systems of values. The scenarios discussed in the first part of this chapter demonstrate that ethics should not only be associated with dramatic and high profile cases; ordinary, even apparently trivial, cases raise important ethical concerns. This is partly because issues are rarely trivial to the people involved, and partly because the same fundamental debates about philosophy or principle underpin routine as well as exceptional decisions. This is why we cannot afford to see ethics as an esoteric concern for the interested few.

In the end, ethical judgement is practical judgement founded on experience and close attention to detail. But this is not to say that it is merely common sense or pragmatism. Ethical judgement has to be informed by some vision of what is going on. What are our conceptions of the good, both for those immediately affected and for the wider society? What are the weaknesses of our conceptions; what are the dangers in doing what we favour? Above all, can we explain and defend the reasons we have for making the decisions we do? Critical reflection on questions like 'what is health?' and 'what is health promotion?' is part of that process. It is complex, and it sometimes threatens ideas or habits with which we are comfortable, but it is the only way we can really call our practice our own. It is the only way we can be truly accountable for what we do.

References

Rowe, K. & Macleod Clark, J. (1993) The coronary care nurse's role in smoking cessation. In *Research in Health Promotion and Nursing* (Eds J.Wilson Barnett & J. Macleod Clark). Macmillan Press, London.

Walsh, P.N. (1988) Handicapped and female: Two disabilities? In *Concepts and Controversies in Services for People with a Mental Handicap.* (Eds N. McConkey & A. McGinley). Woodland Centre, Galway, Ireland.

Voysey, F. (1993) Women's world. *Nursing Times* January 6, **89** (1) 36–8.

Further reading

Beauchamp, T. Childress, J. (1989) *Principles of Biomedical Ethics.* 3rd Ed. Oxford University Press, Oxford.

Downie, R.S., Fyfe, C. and Tannahill, A. (1990) *Health Promotion Models and Values*. Oxford University Press, Oxford.

Doxiadis, S. (Ed.) (1987) *Ethical Dilemmas in Health Promotion*. John Wiley and Sons Ltd, Chichester.

Doxiadis, S. (Ed.) (1990) *Ethics in health education*. John Wiley and Sons Ltd, Chichester.

Part Two
Health Promotion: Practice

Chapter 5

Case Studies of Health Promotion with Adults: Nurses Working with People Who Wish to Stop Smoking

Introduction

The Government's White Paper about health promotion, *The Health of the Nation*, recognizes that hospitals 'offer unique opportunities for ... health promotion for patients, staff and all who come into contact with them'. In addition, the 'special role' of health professionals is acknowledged: 'their opportunities to help and advise individuals, families and communities are unparalleled; (Department of Health, 1992, p. 27, 30).

The White Paper identifies five key areas for action to improve the health of the nation: coronary heart disease and stroke, cancers, mental illness, HIV, AIDS and sexual health, and accidents. One contribution towards combating the first three is that there should be a 'high priority given to the provision of advice on smoking and support for those wishing to stop' (Department of Health, 1992, p. 78). This chapter examines health promotion with adults by considering two case studies of smoking cessation.

In Great Britain 32% of the population smoke cigarettes (Department of Health, 1991). Smoking is associated with many health problems, from lung cancer and heart disease to chronic bronchitis and low birthweight babies. Nurses, in their detailed work with patients, are well placed to help those wishing to stop smoking. Until recently, however, the most effective ways of doing this were unclear. Now some important research has started to emerge which begins to indicate how this goal might best be achieved. This chapter discusses this research, indicating how nurses might more usefully function in this area of health promotion.

Health costs associated with smoking

'It has been estimated that among an average 1000 young adults who smoke cigarettes regularly, about one will be murdered, about six will be killed on the roads, but about 250 will be killed before their time by tobacco' (Department of Health, 1992, p. 70). Cigarette smoking causes about 30% of all cancer deaths. Of this 26 000 a year are from lung cancer and the remainder are from cancers of the mouth, pharynx, larynx, oesophagus, pancreas, bladder and other organs. Cigarette smoking causes 18% of coronary heart disease deaths and up to 11% of stroke deaths. Smoking also contributes to chronic respiratory disease and other health problems.

Smoking in pregnancy is associated with low birthweight and also with a 28% increase in perinatal mortality in babies. Smoking has also been linked with delayed physical and mental development in children and increased risk of ectopic pregnancy. The consequences of the latter for the mother can be severe or even life threatening. This knowledge is of particular concern given that in 1990 more 16–19 year old women smoked than did men of the same age. Passive smoking of environmental tobacco smoke may lead to several hundred deaths each year. It has also been linked to respiratory illnesses in infants and young children (Department of Health, 1991, 1992; Mihill 1992).

Smoking has been described as the 'largest single preventable cause of death' (Department of Health, 1991, p. 36). In the targets set for the health of the nation, the government aims to reduce the prevalence of cigarette smoking to no more than 20% by the year 2000 for both men and women. In addition, it is hoped to reduce cigarette consumption by 40%. The target for smoking in pregnancy is that at least 33% of women will stop smoking at the start of their pregnancy by the year 2000. Young people will also be the focus of attention, with the aim of reducing the smoking prevalence of 11–15 year olds by at least 33% by 1994. Given the health costs associated with smoking the question of how nurses might most effectively enable patients to quit smoking becomes of crucial importance.

Helping people who wish to stop smoking

Research focusing exclusively on the *nurse's* role in helping patients and clients to stop smoking was conducted by a team of nurse researchers at The Department of Nursing Studies, King's College, University of London (Macleod Clark *et al.* 1990). The study involved 20 qualified staff who were working as hospital nurses, health visitors or midwives. Participants were invited to attend two one-day workshops.

The first day centred around the effects of smoking and cessation strategies. Debates were also held about theories and models of health

Table 5.1   Framework for health education.

Assessment
Assess the smoker in terms of motivation to give up, health beliefs and fears or worries about continuing to smoke or giving up. Information should relate to the individual's health beliefs.

Planning
Plan a course of action to stop smoking *with* the smoker not *for* him/her. Utilize constructively knowledge of cessation strategies and outside agencies such as smokers' clinics. Suggest coping strategies.

Implementation
Client attempts to implement plan; nurse's role is one of support and encouragement. The nurse can act as referral agent if continued support is impractical.

Evaluation
Evaluate intervention in terms of client attitude and behaviour and your own approach. If plan has failed, look at where it went wrong and start again. Reinforce positive changes in smoking behaviour.

---

education and hospital smoking policies. Before the second day the 20 participants were asked to audio-record themselves talking to someone who wanted to give up smoking. These recordings were used at the workshop for developing the participants' communication skills. Emphasis was placed on effective listening, the use of open questions, the avoidance of closed or leading questions and the use of structure within the intervention. A framework was introduced for smoking health education, based on the nursing process and the health belief model (Becker 1974) – see Table 5.1.

Following the two study days the participating nurses, midwives and health visitors were asked to speak to up to five of their patients or clients about giving up smoking. Sixteen of the participants were able to do this with a total of 68 patients or clients. Conversations about smoking cessation between the two parties were tape recorded. In addition, each patient or client in the study completed a checklist assessing their level of motivation to stop smoking, worries about the health consequences of continued smoking, and the implications of stopping smoking for their health. A Bedfont carbon monoxide monitor was used with all patients and clients as a health education and validation tool. Patients and clients were also followed up at six months and one year to collect any data on changes in smoking behaviour and to ask for recollections and perceptions of the professional's intervention. Urinary cotinine levels were also taken as a validation measure at one year, from patients and clients who had stopped smoking.

Findings of the nurses', health visitors' and midwives' study

At one year follow-up, 17% of the 42 patients who completed the study had stopped smoking. This compares favourably with attempts by other health professionals working in this area. In studies focusing on GPs, for example, between 5% and 15% of patients stopped smoking (Russell *et al.* 1979; Jamrozik *et al.* 1984 and Russell *et al.* 1987). Of the remaining patients and clients in the present study, as can be seen in Table 5.2, 12% had cut down substantially and 31% had made at least one attempt to give up. The remainder had not changed their behaviour at all. Thus 60% of the clients and patients may have been influenced by the nurses', midwives' and health visitors' attempts to help them stop smoking.

Tables 5.2   Change in smoking behaviour at one year follow-up (*n* = 42).

Smoking behaviour	n	%
Stopped smoking	7	17
Cut down substantially	5	12
Made at least one attempt to give up	13	31
No change in behaviour	17	40

The checklist of patients' and clients' worries about smoking revealed a greater concern with breathlessness and lung cancer than heart disease. The sample included a number of young mothers and pregnant women and their concern for the health of their babies and young children was reflected. Table 5.3 gives the full results.

The focus on breathlessness may demonstrate a preoccupation with the more immediate health costs associated with smoking rather than a concern with more long-term dangers. This links with the idea of 'functional ability' – being able to perform the activities of daily living – which has been found to be an important part of lay conceptions of health (Williams, 1983; Blaxter, 1987). The greater anxiety about lung

Table 5.3   Beliefs and worries about the effects of smoking.

	%	n
Effects on health of baby	68.5	47
Breathlessness	66.7	45
Lung cancer	66.6	45
Heart disease	59.2	40
Effects on health of family	57.4	39

cancer rather than heart disease may reflect a belief in cancer as the incurable disease, the disease to be dreaded (Blaxter, 1983).

Questioning about the implications of stopping smoking for the patients' and clients' health revealed that the majority expected to feel a sense of achievement (81.4%) and to experience greater physical fitness (76.9%) if they successfully quitted. Concerns about weight gain (70.3%) and feelings of irritability (66.6%) were also expressed. Psychological phenomena such as a feeling of happiness and an absence of stress and worry have been shown to be central to a person's own health assessment (Blaxter, 1987). The threat that quitting smoking poses to this may prove to be an important barrier to successful cessation. Patients and clients will need to address this and, with the support of the nurse, devise coping strategies if they are to achieve their goal.

Analysis of the tape-recorded conversations revealed that most were between 10 and 20 minutes in length. In the majority (58%) of cases the professionals did more talking than the patient or client exercising considerable 'control' over the conversation. In 21% of cases the client or patient talked more than the professional and in the remaining 21% the balance was more equal.

The transcripts were also analysed to explore the use of the health education framework. In general, the nurses, midwives and health visitors were able to make a fairly detailed *assessment* of the client as suggested by the framework for health education. Sometimes, however, they were not able to discover the true level of motivation of the client, although some transcripts did show the professionals helping to raise the client's level of motivation. The second *planning* phase of the framework proved more problematic. There was a tendency to fall back on prescriptive advice, telling the client what was 'best', not focusing on the client's needs or helping them to think through what might work best for them.

One or two clients who were strongly motivated to stop did participate to some extent in working out a cessation strategy. The hospital nurses found difficult the support required in the *implementation* phase as they did not normally have the opportunity to see patients again; one nurse however, did telephone a patient to see how he was getting on. The health visitors and midwives, in contrast, found this easier because of the long term nature of their relationships with clients.

A very interesting finding emerged when the outcome of the nurse's intervention was compared with the way in which she had attempted the health education. There did appear to be a relationship between the use of open questions, listening and positive response to cues, and the successful outcome in terms of smoking cessation. In addition, the more successful attempts at health education were those where the patient or client was involved in the planning process, particularly those where there was a high ratio of client/patient talk to professional talk. It seems the full participation of the client in the interaction is a hallmark of success. This research was based on a small sample, but this finding does point the way forward for some intriguing further research and may help us see how nurses might be more effective in this area of health promotion.

From this study, given the predominance of very real concerns about increased stress and weight gain when stopping smoking, it is clear that any successful attempt to help people will need to address these negative effects and devise coping strategies. Other research by Calnan and Williams (1991) reinforces the importance of viewing smoking in the context of lay health beliefs. Gender differences about the social meaning of smoking emerged in their study; the relaxing and stress-relieving nature of smoking was expressed by all the women who smoked. Men, in contrast, emphasized the habitual and sociable nature of smoking. This understanding might be used by nurses helping patients to devise appropriate coping strategies.

A significant relationship also, perhaps predictably, emerged from the study of the client's or patient's confidence and motivation to give up smoking, compared with their subsequent success. This suggests that a more effective use of health care resources might be to focus health education about cessation on those truly motivated to stop, while attempting to enhance the remainder's motivation rather than discuss cessation. Assessment emerged as having a crucial part to play in identifying these two groups of smokers. In retrospect it is clear that many patients or clients were not really strongly motivated to give up, even though at the outset of the intervention they had claimed to be so.

Cornwell (1984) in her study of lay health beliefs identified the importance of 'public' and 'private' accounts when speaking about matters of health and illness. Public accounts focus on widely acceptable views that are likely to gain the approval of the listener. In the health context 'they exclude experiences and opinions that might be considered unacceptable to members of the medical profession'. Private accounts are shared once an interviewer is 'accepted', and they tend to be anecdotal, discussing experiences by reference to 'material concerns and practical constraints that intrude into matters of health and illness'. Here medically unacceptable values and opinions are stated. The use of effective communication skills within a non-judgemental atmosphere might also enable nurses, midwives and health visitors to move from public to more private accounts in their health promotion work.

How coronary care nurses might help patients wanting to give up smoking

More recently a second study has developed the original research (Rowe & Macleod Clark, 1993). Building on the earlier findings, the second study continued to shape the health education intervention to the individual patient or client. In addition, in line with the earlier research, only patients who were highly motivated to stop smoking were included in the programme. The patients were encouraged to participate fully in the intervention and were also offered long term support.

The research took place in a coronary care unit and involved patients with severe angina or first time myocardial infarction. All patients who expressed a desire to stop smoking were invited to take part in an individualized smoking cessation programme. Ten patients joined, and a reference group of a further ten patients, who did not participate in the research but received 'standard' advice, were also identified. These were matched as far as possible to the patients participating in the smoking cessation programme.

The second study utilized a similar framework for health education to that used in the earlier research. The *assessment* phase took place in the coronary care unit as soon as appropriate after admission. It consisted of the patient filling in a motivation checklist and the nurse conducting an interview. The motivation checklist, which was completed before the interview, indicated the patient's desire to stop smoking and his determination and confidence to do so. This knowledge enabled the nurse to identify any problem areas. The tape-recorded interview followed a semi-structured approach incorporating open and closed questions. This allowed in-depth knowledge to be gained about the individual patient, allowing for probing and response to non-verbal cues. Smoking behaviour, health beliefs and degree of motivation to stop smoking were also explored during the interview.

An individualized smoking cessation intervention was then *planned* with the patient. After identification of needs, coping strategies were discussed with the patient, planning which strategy best suited him. The importance of encouraging participation in this process had been identified in the earlier study. As a result it was felt vital that the patient himself, with the aid of the nurse, explored potential problems with smoking cessation and strategies for overcoming them. Patients were also encouraged to think and talk about the possible relationship between their smoking behaviour and admission to hospital with coronary heart disease.

In line with the *implementation* phase of the health education

Health Promotion

framework, a support programme was offered to the patients. A telephone call was made on a weekly or monthly basis as desired by the patient. All patients were also aware they could telephone whenever they were experiencing a problem. Once again the significance of support had been identified by the earlier research.

Evaluation of the programme consisted of following up the patients in their own homes at six months, 12 months and 24 months. At this time experiences of trying to change smoking behaviour were monitored, support was offered and encouragement and further advice given if required. A checklist provided useful information on smoking behaviour since discharge and assessed how the intervention itself was perceived.

Carbon monoxide levels were measured using a Bedfont CO_2 monitor. This provided both a source of encouragement to the patients and a confirmation of self-reported smoking behaviour. Those patients whose partners or families smoked tended to have higher levels of carbon monoxide in their expired air, from passive smoking. Thus the exercise also served an educational purpose. Salivary samples for cotinine levels were also collected to confirm smoking behaviour.

Findings of the coronary care nurses' study

Of the patients participating in the study, 77% were successful in stopping smoking at six months, 77% at one year and 75% at two years (see Table 5.4). These results compare favourably with a study by Taylor *et al.* (1990) where cessation rates at one year, in a nurse-managed intervention for first-time myocardial infarction patients, were 61% for the intervention group and 32% for the usual care group. All successful patients in the present study had been diagnosed as suffering a myocardial infarction (MI). One of these patients died prior to the two year follow-up. However, at one year follow up he had said: 'I feel so well, so healthy, I'm a new man. I wish I'd stopped years ago.'

The two patients in the research group who were diagnosed as suffering from angina continued to smoke throughout the two years. Both had relapsed before six months – at three and eleven weeks. Following support and encouragement both had tried again and were successful in reducing their cigarette consumption by 40% and 50%. The other patient who did not quit smoking cut down his cigarette consumption but dropped out of the study at three months. All three clients within the research group who continued to smoke had experienced emotional disturbances: two were now widowed and one unemployed.

Those patients in the research group who stopped smoking were found to differ in certain respects from those who did not cease at six months. These differences included their medical diagnosis, length of

Table 5.4 Evaluation of the smoking cessation programme.

Research group	6 months	1 year	2 years
MI – not smoking	77% ($n = 7$)	77% ($n = 7$)	75% ($n = 6$)
			One died at 18 months
MI – smoking	0% ($n = 0$)	0% ($n = 0$)	0% ($n = 0$)
Angina – not smoking	0% ($n = 0$)	0% ($n = 0$)	0% ($n = 0$)
Angina – smoking	23% ($n = 2$)	23% ($n = 2$)	25% ($n = 2$)
	One withdrew from study		
Totals	100% ($n = 9$)	100% ($n = 9$)	100% ($n = 8$)
Reference group			
MI – smoking	30% ($n = 3$)	17% ($n = 1$)	—
		Two deaths at seven months	
Angina – smoking	70% ($n = 7$)	83% ($n = 6$)	—
		One death at nine months	
Totals	100% ($n = 10$)	100% ($n = 7$)	—

stay in hospital, previous cardiac history and previous cardiac admissions. All seven patients who stopped smoking at six months had a myocardial infarction and were in hospital from seven to nine days. Only one patient had a previous cardiac history and two had previous cardiac admissions. All patients who did not stop smoking had a diagnosis of angina and each had a previous cardiac history. In total the research group had seven previous cardiac admissions compared to a total of 49 for the reference group.

The motivational checklist used as part of the initial *assessment* phase asked three questions to assess the patients' commitment to stopping smoking:

(1) *Desire* How much do you want to give up smoking?
(2) *Determination* How determined are you to give up smoking?
(3) *Confidence* How sure are you that if you tried you would give up smoking?

The results are given in Table 5.5 and demonstrate higher levels of desire, determination and confidence in giving up smoking in the research group than the reference group. The interview transcripts were also used to identify any differences in motivation between those who gave up smoking and those who did not. All the patients who successfully stopped smoking had said in their interview that they were strongly

Table 5.5 Motivation to give up smoking.

	Research group	Reference group
Desire		
I want to very much	8 (80%)	0 (0%)
I would like to	2 (20%)	2 (20%)
I don't know	0 (0%)	5 (50%)
I don't really want to	0 (0%)	3 (30%)
I don't want to at all	0 (0%)	0 (0%)
Determination		
I am very determined	7 (70%)	0 (0%)
I am fairly determined	3 (30%)	2 (20%)
Neither	0 (0%)	7 (70%)
I am fairly undetermined	0 (0%)	0 (0%)
I am not determined	0 (0%)	1 (10%)
Confidence		
I am very sure that if I tried I could give up	3 (30%)	0 (0%)
I am fairly sure	4 (40%)	0 (0%)
I don't know	3 (30%)	8 (80%)
I am fairly unsure	0 (0%)	1 (10%)
I am very unsure	0 (0%)	1 (10%)

motivated, for example: 'I definitely want to give up smoking' and 'I'd love to quit them altogether'.

Exploration of the patients' health beliefs demonstrated that all ten patients in the research group associated smoking with heart disease and 70% made a causative link with lung cancer. All ten patients also expected to experience a sense of achievement if they gave up smoking.

Examination of the interview transcripts, shown in Table 5.6, also demonstrates how some patients had clearly made a strong link in their minds between smoking and coronary heart disease. This contrasts with the findings in the earlier study where heart disease was seen as less important as a health consequence of smoking than breathlessness and lung cancer. As we might expect, the immediacy of the acute coronary heart disease would appear to be of prime importance.

In the *planning* phase of the programme, a range of coping strategies were identified by the patients. These ranged from oral substitution, diversion activity and recalling the experience of the myocardial infarction. All subjects who had had a myocardial infarction were able to identify positive behavioural and cognitive self-support mechanisms. All seven patients who were successful in maintaining smoking cessation were able to recall their coping strategies at the six month follow-up visit.

If ever I'm tempted, I'll just think back to that pain in that store. That's the one thing I would think back to. I will never forget it.'

These views support the idea that being prepared for a problem makes coping easier and so reduces the likelihood of relapse.

With regard to *implementation*, there was a high level of desire for further support expressed by the patients. All those who experienced a myocardial infarction requested a telephone link. Two clients who did not cease smoking did not have the facility of a telephone so requested a visit. Nine (90%) of the subjects found the interview helpful. Only one subject did not express any need of help. Interestingly this patient withdrew from the study at three months. The programme appears to have been most effective in the way it enabled patients to identify and use coping strategies, and build up patients' confidence levels and offered ongoing support.

Previous studies have suggested that the experience of having a myocardial infarction may provide the strongest motivation to stop smoking, even without any specific intervention (Hoy & Turbott, 1970; Wilhelmsson *et al.*, 1975; Croog & Richards, 1977; Sparrow *et al.*, 1978; Sivarajan *et al.* 1983). This study, however, found that the majority of patients (90%) expressed a positive desire for support. The individual nursing intervention provided the means whereby this support could be given.

As was implicitly recognized in the Health of the Nation document, a stay in hospital provides a prime opportunity to encourage non-smoking.

Table 5.6 Views of the link between coronary heart disease and smoking, by patients who stopped smoking.

Patient no.	Answers to question 'Why do you want to give up smoking?
(1)	I got a real fright. The 'lights' were on the dim for me that Friday. They could have been switched out just as easy as that ... Cigarettes did that.
(3)	Its essential for my health ... I must stop smoking ... I'll be dead if I don't.
(4)	This heart attack has made me want to give up smoking. Look what cigarettes have done ... I slipped away you know.
(5)	Look what they've done to my heart.
(7)	Having this heart attack has brought it home to me that smoking does affect your health.
(9)	Definitely cigarettes have caused this ... look, I even had a cigarette in my hand when it happened.
(10)	Well, I've had a heart attack and if cigarettes can do that to me I've got to take this chance now. I could have died that day.

To determine why some of the patients were more successful than others in stopping smoking, the length of stay in hospital was considered. It was found that all seven patients (70%) who had stopped smoking were hospitalized for seven to nine days, while the remaining three (30%) who cut down their cigarette consumption were only in hospital for two to three days. Length of stay did indeed seem to be an important factor, possibly because it provided an opportunity for maximum support and encouragement in the initial stages of smoking cessation. Nine (90%) of the subjects made reference to this fact at some stage during the study: 'Having help is a great opportunity'.

The research indicated that patients who experience their first myocardial infarction appear more likely to accept the link between smoking behaviour and coronary heart disease than those with severe angina and a long cardiac history. The intervention was found to be feasible in terms of nursing time, and cost effective because of the lower re-admission rate of clients who stopped smoking. In this study, nine of the ten interventions were carried out by the research nurse, unit nursing staff feeling ill equipped to do so. Interestingly, the one patient who was interviewed by a nurse from the unit maintained smoking cessation at two years. Previous research has also shown nurses unable or reluctant to fulfil this particular health education function (Haverty *et al.* 1986; Latter *et al.*, 1992). In order that all nurses might fulfil this role in future it appears that further education will be needed to enhance nurses' communication skills and equip them with greater knowledge of the health impact of smoking and cessation strategies.

How nurses might help patients to stop smoking

From these two pieces of research we now have a slightly clearer picture of how nurses might best help patients wishing to give up smoking. More detailed and larger scale research is however still very much needed. The indications from this work suggest that we should focus cessation programmes on those who actually want to give up smoking. For the remainder of patients who are not motivated to quit, we need to discover ways of enhancing their motivation rather than perhaps misguidedly recruiting them to cessation programmes.

A hallmark of success in helping people to stop smoking appears to be that patients should be encouraged to participate fully in the programme rather than being merely the passive recipient of prescriptive advice. Encouraging participation has the added advantage that we demonstrate respect for the patient as a person, rather than making him the subject of our paternalistic judgements. (For a more detailed discussion of the ethical issues raised by smoking cessation see Chapter 4.) By facilitating participation, through the effective use of communication skills, we may stimulate the patient to think about his own coping strategies, both cognitive and behavioural. It also seems that patients attempting to quit smoking would like support in this endeavour and find the nurse an acceptable figure to fulfil this role.

For nurses working in the specialized environment of a coronary care unit, there is some evidence that focusing on patients who have been admitted with a first time myocardial infarction might be beneficial. In addition, patients involved in a stop smoking programme might benefit from being encouraged to think and talk about any link they see between their experience of coronary heart disease and their smoking. There may also be a case for seeking longer stays in hospital as a means to more effectively establish smoking cessation. In economic terms this might be justified in terms of reduced recurrence rates. Finally, it seems that before being able to effectively fulfil this function as nurses, we will need to be further educated about the health consequences of smoking, cessation strategies and frameworks and communication skills.

In thinking more generally about the nurse's role in helping people to stop smoking, it should be noted that the work reviewed in this chapter has focused exclusively on work with individuals. To use the terms of the Ottawa Charter for Health (WHO, 1986, see also Chapter 2), the work has primarily been concerned to 'develop the personal skills' of the patients who wished to stop smoking through the 'creation of a supportive environment'. For the health practitioner, the adoption of the smoking cessation programme is an example of 'building healthy public policy' at the micro level of the hospital ward or community health care. The attempts at working in partnership with the patients and clients and encouraging effective participation in the process are a small step to 'reorienting health services'.

Making the choice of not smoking easier

In addition to this fairly individual approach, health promotion is about making healthy choices easier choices in a broader sense. In this way, as nurses, we may have additional, less direct but no less important, roles to play in helping patients to stop smoking. In the White Paper about health promotion, the government recognizes that 'in the end, the decision of whether or not to smoke is a matter of individual choice, although *this is influenced by many factors*' [our italics]. (Department of Health, 1992).

The document then discusses the impact, for example, of the price of

cigarettes, controls on smoking in public places and controls on advertising and promotion. Collectively, we may attempt to influence these
factors through our professional organizations. The Royal College of
Nursing is pressing for increased taxation on cigarettes and tobacco,
stricter limitations on advertising, the end of sports sponsorship, universal penalties for those selling cigarettes to children under 16 and the
extension of a smoke-free environment (Royal College of Nursing, 1991).
It may be that, individually we should be lobbying for these changes by
writing to our local MP, becoming involved with local government,
organizing boycotts of sporting events where tobacco products are
promoted and visiting local employers to encourage the provision of
smoke-free places of work in our local communities.

These ideas may seem rather idealistic or perhaps too political for
some people. Others might see them as falling naturally within a nurse's
attempt to influence policies which affect health, thereby indirectly
helping people to stop smoking or not take up the habit in the first place.
Once again, to adopt the language of the Ottawa Charter, these are
examples of nurses working collectively and individually to try to build
'healthy public policy'.

Constraints on people's choices about smoking

In working towards helping people to stop smoking other aspects of the
social context, not explicitly addressed in the White Paper, need to be
borne in mind. Graham (1989) has shown how there are strong barriers
that make it very difficult for some women to choose not to smoke; for
women on low incomes smoking is an important coping mechanism:

> 'I think smoking stops me getting irritable, I can cope with things
> better. If I was economizing, I'd cut down on cigarettes but I wouldn't
> give up. I'd stop eating. That sounds terrible doesn't it? Food just isn't
> that important to me but having a cigarette is the only thing I do just
> for myself.'

> (Lone mother)

For women like this, health promotion might usefully address their poor
housing, financial difficulties, relentless childcare duties or their low self
esteem. A health visitor might work with similar women trying to
empower them so that they might influence the local council to improve
their housing facilities, or lobby Parliament for improved financial help
for single parent families. Alternatively, she might try to work with the

women to develop their personal skills so that they can organize and run their own crèche facilities. Raising the women's self esteem through group work might enable them to identify other things they could do 'just for themselves' instead of smoking.

In addressing the question of housing and financial support the health visitor is contributing to a 'reorientation of health services' in directing action towards these determinants of health. In so doing she also involves herself in 'building healthy public policy'. By attempting to develop the personal skills of the women to lobby the local council and their MP and by working with them to run a crèche, she is strengthening community action and helping them to create a more supportive environment for themselves.

An awareness of the social context of smoking also highlights other ways in which people are not entirely free agents with regard to their smoking behaviour. Men and women in the semi-skilled and unskilled socio-economic groups are much more likely to smoke than those in the remaining groups (Central Statistical Office, 1993). Rodmell & Watt (1986), writing about a social group's lifestyle, say: 'It is useful to understand it as representing a set of practices established over time and over which people *do not necessarily have control* [our italics]'.

Bearing this in mind, as nurses working towards helping people to stop smoking, we need to tread a fine balance between facilitating the healthy choice of no smoking and at the same time not falling prey to either victim blaming or healthism. Holding people entirely responsible for their continued smoking or failure to quit may be an example of victim blaming with its lack of recognition that although 'the decision of whether or not to smoke is a matter of individual choice ... *this is influenced by many factors* [our italics]' (Department of Health, 1992).

Similarly, criticism of people who choose to continue to smoke because they enjoy it, despite being aware of the health consequences, may be an example of healthism with its assumption that health should be valued *above all else* by all human beings. Such a view may fail to respect a person's right to choose, even if the choice is health damaging.

Conclusion

This chapter has explored how nurses might work with people who wish to stop smoking, as two case studies of health promotion with adults. The focus has mainly been on primary and tertiary preventive health education by hospital nurses. Helping people to stop smoking is only one part of health promotion in this area. Working towards a society where people do not start smoking in the first place is another major focus. All nurses, not just those in acute hospital settings, may have a part to play in these aspects of health promotion. School nurses have an important role with young people. Health visitors may be involved in their work with the whole family and community. Practice nurses will be involved in their work in the surgery, especially with their responsibilities in smoking cessation clinics. Occupational health nurses have a key role to play in the workplace. Midwives have a unique opportunity to help pregnant women to stop smoking. Community psychiatric nurses and nurses working with those with learning disabilities may also have some input. More research is needed to help us understand how we may more effectively work in this area. The studies discussed in this chapter are important steps in this process of discovery.

References

Becker, M.H. (1974). The Health Belief Model and Personal Health Behaviour. *Health Education Monographs*, 2, 324–508.

Blaxter, M. (1983) The causes of disease. Women talking. *Social Science and Medicine* **17** , (2) 59–69.

Blaxter, M. (1987) Attitudes to Health. in *The Health and Lifestyle Survey*. (Eds Cox, B., Blaxter, M., Buckle, A.L.J., Fenner, N.P., Golding, J.F., Gore, M., Huppery, F.A., Nickson, J., Roth, M., Stark, J., Wadsworth, M.E.J. and Whichelow, M.) Health Promotion Research Trust, London.

Calnan, M. & Williams, S. (1991) Style of life and the salience of health: an exploratory study of health related practices in households from differing socio-economic circumstances. *Sociology of health and illness.* **13** (4) 506–29.

Central Statistical Office (1993) *Social Trends*, 23. Her Majesty's Stationery Office, London.

Cornwell, J. (1984) *Hard earned lives*. Tavistock, London.

Croog, S.H., & Richards, N.P. (1977) Health beliefs and smoking patterns in heart patients and their wives. A longitudinal study. *American Journal Public Health*. **67**, 921–30.

Department of Health (1991) *The Health of the Nation*. Her Majesty's Stationery Office, London.

Department of Health (1992) *The Health of the Nation*. Her Majesty's Stationery Office, London.

Graham, H. (1989) The changing patterns of women's smoking. *Health Visitor*. January, **62** 2–24.

Haverty, S., Macleod Clark, J., & Kendall, S. (1986) Nurses and smoking education: a literature review. *Nurse Education Today*, **6**, 237–43.

Hoy, D.R., & Turbett, S. (1970) Changes in smoking habits in the man under 65 years after myocardial infarction and coronary insufficiency. *British Heart Journal*, 32, 738–40.

Jamrozik, K., Fowler, G., Vessey, M. Wald, N., Parker, G., & Van Vunakis, H. (1984) Controlled trials of three different anti-smoking interventions in general practice. *British Medical Journal*, 288, 1499–1515.

Latter, S., Macleod Clark, J., Wilson-Barnett, J. & Maben, J. (1992) Health education in nursing: perceptions of practice in acute settings. *Journal of Advanced Nursing*, 17, 164–72.

Macleod Clark, J., Haverty, S., & Kendall, S. (1990) Helping people to stop smoking: a study of the nurse's role. *Journal of Advanced Nursing*, **16**, 357–63.

Mihill, C. (1992) Waldegrave turns up the heat on smokers. *The Guardian*, 20 February.

Rodmell, S. & Watt, A (1986) Conventional Health Education; Problems and Possibilities. In *The Politics of Health Education – Raising the Issues*. (Eds Rodmell, S. & Watt, A.) (1986). Routledge and Kegan Paul Ltd, London.

Rowe, K. and Macleod Clark, J. (1993) The coronary care nurse's role in smoking cessation. In *Research in Health Promotion and Nursing* (Eds Wilson Barnett, J. & Macleod Clark, J.) (1993). Macmillan Press, London.

Royal College of Nursing (1991) *A Manifesto for Health*. RCN, London.

Russell, M.A.H., Wilson, C., Taylor, C. & Baker, C.D. (1979) The effect of general practitioners advice against smoking. *British Medical Journal*, 28 July, 231–5.

Russell, M.A.H., Stapleton, J.A., Jackson, P.H., Hajek, P. and Becker, M. (1987) District programme to reduce smoking: effect of clinic supported brief intervention by general practitioners. *British Medical Journal*, **291** 1240–4.

Sivarajan, E.S., Newton, K.M., Almes, M.J. (1983) Limited effects of outpatient teaching and counselling after myocardial infarction: a controlled study. *Heart Lung* **12**, 65–73.

Sparrow, D., Dawber, T.R. & Colton, T (1978) The influence of cigarette smoking after a first myocardial infarction. *Journal of Chronic Disability*, **31**, 425–32.

Taylor, C.B., Houston-Miller, N., Killen, J.D. & DeBusk, R.F. (1990) Smoking cessation after acute myocardial infarction: effects of a nurse-managed intervention. *Annuals of Internal Medicine*. **113**, 118–23.

WHO (1986) *Ottawa Charter for Health Promotion*. World Health Organization & Health and Welfare, Ottawa, Canada.

Wilhelmsson, C., Vedin, J.A., Elmfeldt, D., Tibblin, G. & Wilhelmsen, L. (1975) Smoking and myocardial infarction. *The Lancet*, 22 February.

Williams, R. (1983) Concepts of health: an analysis of lay logic. *Sociology* **17**, 2, 185–205.

Chapter 6
Health Promotion, School Nursing and the School Age Child

In the first few terms at school, children will be taught to read, write and count. But they will also learn about behaviour in a group: how to respond to peers, and how to relate to adults who are not their parents or minders.

As a child moves towards adulthood there will be rapid physical development and there will also be a shift in attitudes and values. 'Sensible' attitudes previously held on such matters as smoking and the use of alcohol may be reversed; the need to conform to their social or peer groups develops strongly. Thus school-age children are not only open to positive educational influence but are also vulnerable to external pressures at a time when habits may be acquired which will last a lifetime. For these reasons this group should not only have access to information on health and healthy lifestyles but they must be guided through this challenging time and helped to make healthy choices, often in the face of unfavourable extrinsic pressures. Health must be a positive motivating force in their lives.

Educational context

Section 1 of the 1988 Education Reform Act places statutory responsibility on schools to provide a broad and balanced curriculum which:

(1) promotes the spiritual, moral, cultural, mental and physical development of pupils at the school and of society;
(2) prepares pupils for the opportunities, responsibilities and experiences of adult life

National Curriculum Council Guidance Document No. 3

The national curriculum sets specific programmes of study. Schools are bound by statute to cover all the attainment targets within the programmes in the nine core subjects. There are also a number of guidance documents which are part of the national curriculum but are not a legal requirement. National Curriculum Council Guidance Document 5 relates to health education and covers the components for a health education curriculum for children between five and sixteen years. How far these are incorporated into the main subjects depends on the school's commitment to health education.

Constraints

In addition to there being no compulsion for schools to include a thorough health programme, there are a number of other constraints which lead to a low profile for health education within the core subjects.

Teachers are under enormous pressure to cover all the areas outlined in the national curriculum. Children are now undergoing tests at specific ages and the results of these tests are being used as a measure of success of the academic programme. This is becoming an even greater issue because parents will have access to the results and will be able to apply for a place for their child at the school of their choice. Now that the schools have a responsibility to maintain their own budget there is competition between schools to ensure a full roll in order to secure the maximum amount of finance. As a consequence, there is enormous emphasis on academic achievement as measured by the published tests. This is an important influence as far as the nine core subjects are concerned, and is a disadvantage for other subjects such as health education.

Inevitably, the inclusion of health education in the education programme is dependent on the school's commitment to health. But surely it makes sense to assist schoolchildren so that they can acquire the life skills and knowledge vital to their physical and mental health and to develop a positive self-image and self-esteem. An excellent academic education will be a poor investment in a child that develops unhealthy habits, is physically unfit and emotionally vulnerable.

Even if a school does possess a positive philosophy towards health, it is important that teachers have the skills required to deliver the information which imparts knowledge to children, assists them in learning how to make healthy choices and equips them with the confidence to say no. Some health education topics are relatively easy to teach children, for example, nutrition. There are some extremely good resources available and because children relate well to the subject matter, learning is both enjoyable and applicable. Children tend to be aware of the difference between healthy and unhealthy food and a good teaching programme will assist them in making healthy choices.

Other subjects are more complex and include more conspicuous moral and ethical dilemmas. Personal and social education (including sex education) present teachers with many difficulties. First, teachers may be constrained by their personal attitudes and values. Equally, a class of thirty children may include a number of different religions and cultures where some information and discussions would be acceptable to some but not all.

Sex education is the one area of health education which is covered by statute. For county, controlled and maintained special schools, section 18(2) of the Education (No. 2) Act 1986 requires that:

'The articles of government for every such school shall provide for it to be the duty of the governing body:

(a) to consider separately (while having regard to the Local Education Authority's statement under Section 17 of this Act on their policy in relation to the secular curriculum in maintained schools) the question whether sex education should form part of the secular curriculum for the school; and

(b) to make and keep to date, a separate written statement of their policy with regard to the content and organization of the relevant part of the curriculum; or where they conclude that sex education should not form part of the secular curriculum, of that conclusion.

National Curriculum Council Guidance Document No. 5

The Act gave the responsibility to the school governors of deciding on a sex education policy. The policy could simply state that sex education would not be included in the school curriculum. Enlightened schools have developed comprehensive policies and integrated the subject in a carefully planned and adequate programme. There are some primary schools which have had successful programmes running for several years, by contrast some secondary schools have chosen to exclude the topic altogether.

Schools considering developing a health education programme should identify other professionals who may be able to contribute. Members of the school health team, health promotion officers, family planning nurses and dietitians all have a commitment to health education and are particularly interested in targeting young people. Some would be able to participate in the development of a school health policy and others may contribute to the health education sessions directly. It is vital that education and health are brought together in an integrated programme and professionals work together to fulfil the aims and objectives of a school health policy.

Whitehead (1989) describes a health promoting school and emphasizes the need to move away from the traditional style of covering specific and somewhat limited topics at specific ages. Many schools have the talk on menstruation with girls in their last term at primary school. Frequently, this is a single session which bears no relation to anything else being taught and may lead to limited information and unanswered questions. Health education needs to be an integrated and continuous programme available to all pupils throughout the school years (HMSO, 1992).

Teaching about health

A good health education programme must be supported by appropriate teaching skills. Professionals responsible for or involved in health promotion may benefit from additional training. For example, school nurses are qualified nurses who do not automatically undertake courses in order to work with school age children. Individual knowledge and teaching ability should be assessed and courses such as the Certificate in Health Education, the family planning course and a counselling course considered. Nurses who have undertaken the Project 2000 course will have had a preparation for the promotion of health and may find the concept of the health-promoting school easier to comprehend and will contribute more naturally to the requirements of the school population.

Traditionally, school nurses have been employed to work in schools with little if any consideration being given to the needs of the school population. The needs of a rural primary school are very different to those of a large urban secondary school. In the former there is likely to be considerable community spirit and support, families know one another, everyone speaks the same language and possibly follows the same religion. In contrast, the secondary school population will include pupils from many different backgrounds, there will be a variety of languages and dialects spoken and numerous religions will be represented. And there is no doubt that, in general, the needs of adolescents are very different from those of the younger child.

The United Kingdom Central Council (UKCC) is currently reviewing community nurses' education and training. Instead of the disciplines distinct from one another (district nurses, health visitors, school nurses etc.) it seems an ideal time for all community nurses to be taught a basic post-registration course and then to develop the specific skills for a certain population through a modular training system. A nurse wishing to work with adolescents will need skills different from those of a nurse who cares for the terminally ill patient or the elderly. In summary, skills must be attached to need and this applies equally to nurses and teachers.

The health promoting school

A health promoting school takes a wider perspective of health. It bases its commitment to health on a model in which physical, mental and environmental aspects interact and which integrates teaching, health care and other components of school such as school meals and the physical environment. Much of the way children behave appears to be through learned behaviour. They will model their behaviour on their parents and, as they get older, teachers and friends. One example of this is the way in which children speak. Not only will they learn a language; they will also learn a vocabulary and how to use it. Language will be used by some children in a way that is considered articulate and polite; others may use the same language in a way that is considered less desirable. Their influences are what they hear from adults and peers. Applied to other forms of behaviour, it becomes evident that role models have a great impact on children and young adults.

A health-promoting school should aim to provide an example to children of health enhancement in all aspects of its functioning. Within a health-promoting school, pupils are encouraged to participate actively in a wide range of projects relating to health in a holistic sense, to develop their own skills and to explore their beliefs, values and attitudes within safe boundaries.

For example, on average there are three children in a class of thirty with asthma. In most schools an asthmatic child will be treated as an isolated deviation from the norm, allowed to bring medication into the school, and monitored by the school health team. This is a limited response, stigmatizing the child. The health-promoting school would consider the needs of children with asthma and ensure a safe and appropriate environment. School staff would have access to training in the management of asthma, medication would be easily accessible, i.e. in the classroom or in the older child's pocket, and possible triggers would be removed from the environment.

All children would be given the opportunity to learn and talk about asthma and would be encouraged to support their peers who have asthma. The parents would be encouraged to keep the staff informed about changes in medication and would be invited to discuss the management of their child's asthma with the teachers and the school health team. In this way the health-promoting school takes a holistic approach to ensuring children's welfare within the school setting.

Health promotion

Who should be involved

Everyone working within the school environment has a responsibility towards promoting the health of children. This includes all teachers, supervisors, sessional and supply staff and the school health team. The head teacher carries the ultimate responsibility for the welfare of pupils but this responsibility is delegated to anyone in control of individuals or groups of children. It is essential that there is good communication and collaboration between all these personnel.

Historically, the role of the school health team has been routine and task-orientated. There is no national health service programme offered to all school age children and the level of school health service provided varies between health authorities. However, the Health Visitors' Association (1991) has highlighted the potential role of school nurses. Many health authorities have been reviewing their school health services and developing the skill-mix. As a result, school nurses are undertaking greater responsibilities within the school setting.

Where this opportunity to review and develop the role of the school nurse has been grasped, the communication and collaboration between the health and education services has been greatly improved. Routine medical screening has been rationalized and other screening is carried out by teams of school nurses and staff based on the guidance in the Hall report (1991).

The school nurse's skills have been developed to ensure they are capable of competently assessing the health of individuals, identifying their health needs and discussing these with the child, parent and teacher. It is through the identification of need that school nurses can work closely with school staff and develop health promotion programmes accordingly.

How it works

At the beginning of each academic year or each term, the teachers and school nurse should meet to identify health promotion targets and the resources required to achieve these targets, and to decide who could contribute to the teaching.

On occasions, other health professionals contribute to the programme, i.e. the school doctor for information about disease and medical conditions; family planning nurses for specialist information on relationships, family planning and sexually transmitted diseases; community psychiatric nurses for information on substance abuse; and health promotion officers on a wide variety of topics. Well-planned programmes provide the opportunity for the most appropriate people to participate and for effective resources to be used.

Some sessions may take place formally in the classroom as part of the national curriculum. However, there are times when health promotion can be easily incorporated into other activities such as meal times, projects, hobbies and homework, playtime and outings. For example, a school nurse arranged a fitness week with one school and organized aerobic sessions in the playground in addition to classroom work. A class looking at accident prevention was asked to identify areas of safe practice and possible areas of danger within their own home. A school nurse had lunch once a week with children in their school dining room and discussed healthy choices of food, explaining why an apple was nutritionally better than a bowl of apple crumble and custard. In a secondary school, school nurses ran group sessions where youngsters had the opportunity to ask questions, understand terminology and be given information on sexuality and relationships in a secure, private and unthreatening environment.

In addition to giving children information about health and healthy choices, it is also extremely important that they should have easy access to immediate advice and support. Some schools have set up drop-in sessions where pupils may talk to the school nurses in private. Being able to talk to a health professional provides a unique environment for obtaining help and advice and for finding ways of resolving the problems either by involving the parents or seeking further expert advice.

The role of the parent or carer should not be overlooked. It is important that parents are encouraged to participate in, or be informed of, health promotion activities. Indeed, there are times when they benefit from advice and support as much as their children. An effective health promoting school will include all those who are part of that community.

Conclusion

The responsibility for health promotion must be shared. Teachers can expand a child's knowledge of their health and, together with health professionals, they have a responsibility to encourage and promote understanding of, and opportunities for, healthy choices. It is essential for children to have access to a planned, organized and well presented programme of health education. Education and health professionals must unite and work together in order to promote the health of school age children and their families and thereby influence the health of the nation.

Table 6.1 Examples of the health promoting school.

Target	Health Promotion Programme
To reduce smoking prevalence of 11–15 year olds by at least 33% by 1994	(1) To develop and adopt a smoking policy for the school environment. (2) To help pupils understand the effects of nicotine on the body. (3) To encourage pupils to say no to a cigarette. (4) To offer pupils, parents and teachers, information on local smoking cessation groups.
To reduce the overall suicide rate by at least 15% by the year 2000	(1) To include mental health in the personal and social health education programme. (2) To provide easy access to a health professional, i.e. regular 'drop-in' sessions run by a school nurse. (3) To provide education for teachers and parents in their support of young people.
To reduce by at least 50% the rate of conception among the under 16s by the year 2000	(1) To develop and adopt a sex education policy. (2) To ensure professionals have the skills to complete the teaching programme. (3) To provide an appropriate environment for the teaching sessions. (4) To inform parents of the content of the programme. (5) To ensure pupils have easy access to advice and counselling. (6) To inform pupils of other agencies who may be able to offer advice and support.
To reduce the death rate for accidents among children aged under 15 by at least 33% by 2005	(1) Accident prevention will be included at the appropriate stages of the national curriculum. (2) Road safety education will include the Green Cross Code. (3) Parents will have the opportunity of attending sessions on accident prevention. (4) Children will be offered road cycling training.
To halt the year-on-year increase in the incidence of skin cancer by 2005	(1) To include information on over-exposure to the sun's rays within the national curriculum. (2) To educate parents and teachers on the importance of children wearing appropriate clothing as a form of protection against the sun's rays.

References

Hall, D. (1991) *Health for All Children* (The Hall Report). Oxford Medical Publications, Oxford.

Health Visitors' Association (1991) *Project Health: Health Promotion and the Role of the School Nurse in the School Community.* Health Visitors' Association, London.

HMSO (1992) *The Health of the Nation – A Strategy for England.* Her Majesty's Stationery Office, London.

National Curriculum Council (1990) *Curriculum Guidance No. 3 The Whole Curriculum.* National Curriculum Council, York.

National Curriculum Council (1990) *Curriculum Guidance No. 5 Health Education.* National Curriculum Council, York.

Whitehead, M. (1989) *Swimming Upstream: Trends and Prospects in Education for Health.* King Edward's Hospital Fund for London, London.

Chapter 7
Promoting Mental Health

Introduction

A professor of psychiatry described the idea of mental health as 'not a very useful concept'. It was simply an absence of symptoms of mental illness. A clinical psychologist suggested he would need ten days at least to discuss the subject and still would not come up with an adequate definition. Neither of these ways of looking at mental health seems to be of much practical use, but the psychologist, after some thought, added that perhaps it might be something like being able to cope with whatever life throws at you without becoming ill. This does at least seem to provide clues to a practical approach.

Mental health and mental illness

For many years now those parts of the national health service which care for people who are mentally ill have called themselves mental health services. Largely as a result of this, mental health to many people actually means mental illness. Even experienced nurses can sometimes equate mental health with such conditions as schizophrenia or manic depression (Armstrong 1992). This is as illogical as saying that physical health means cancer.

The famous World Health Organization definition of health as 'a complete state of physical, mental and social well-being' has not survived without criticism since it was formulated (Ewles & Simnett, 1985), but it does make two important points. One is that health is to do with well-being, about feeling good about one's self. It is more than just not being ill. And the other is to highlight the interdependence of physical, mental and social health. Health has to do with the state of the whole person and that person's relationships with others.

This is not to say that the physically ill person cannot be mentally healthy, or that the mentally ill person may not have a good, supportive family. But there is much research evidence to show that:

(1) People with life-threatening, disabling or painful physical illness are at risk of becoming depressed.
(2) People who have good social and family relationships recover from depressive illnesses more quickly than others.
(3) People with psychiatric disorders have higher death rates from *physical illness* like heart disease and cancers than others (Jenkins & Shepherd, 1983).

While this does not get us any nearer a comprehensive definition of mental health, it does provide some more clues as to what might be meant by *promoting* mental health.

There are practical implications here for nurses and others. First, mental health promotion is part of health promotion in general. It is not something separate to be practised from mental health centres only by specialists. Second, like physical health and illness, mental health and illness may be seen as different sides of the same coin. Knowledge of the effects of smoking gives us reasons for helping people to give up. Knowledge of the factors involved in, say, depression, can similarly provide the justification for helping people develop more effective ways of dealing with their problems. As well as being of therapeutic benefit, this might also be preventative. Third, a commitment to high quality health care means concern for the whole person. In any assessment of health status, questions about mental state are as important as measuring blood pressure.

The analogy with physical health can be taken a stage further. For the non-specialist nurse, that is the nurse without formal training in psychiatry, there are three main aspects to the promotion of mental health in practice:

(1) *The prevention of mental illness* This is likely to be the most problematic area, but there have been suggested strategies around for many years and Newton (1992) considers that we have enough knowledge to begin to put some of it into practice. Secondary and tertiary prevention – for example the prevention of relapse in people with chronic schizophrenia – is largely the province of the specialist practitioner. Primary prevention involves the whole profession.

(2) *The early detection of mental health problems* It is well documented that GPs recognize only about a third of the psychological

problems which present in the general practice surgery (e.g. Goldberg & Huxley, 1980). There is also evidence that those who are recognized get better more quickly than those who are not (Blacker & Clare, 1987). However, GPs do not carry the work of primary health care on their own. Though diagnosis of depression is not always easy, there are relatively simple ways in which nurses can learn to recognize the problem, and alert the GP.

(3) *Mental Health Education* A considerable stigma still attaches to mental illness, much of which probably has to do with deep-seated fears of madness, and guilt associated with being unable to cope. Health education needs to be directed towards enabling people to talk about these fears more openly, and to be more ready to discuss feelings as well as physical symptoms. Health education materials related to mental health are not always easily available from health promotion units. At present little is produced on this subject by the Health Education Authority. However, there are other sources around; a list is given at the end of this chapter. Wider dissemination of such literature could help to make mental health issues more familiar and less frightening.

A few years ago no-one mentioned condoms in polite conversation. Health education campaigns about AIDS have ensured that they are now a common subject for discussion. Mental Health deserves the same kind of attention.

The health of the nation

In 1992 the Government published its White Paper, *Health of the Nation* (HMSO, 1992), setting out a strategy for improvements to the health of people in England in five key areas, of which mental health was one. The need for continuing improvements in treatment, care and rehabilitation is acknowledged, but the document particularly emphasizes disease prevention and health promotion.

A series of targets are set for improvements in various health indicators, most of which are to be achieved by the year 2000.

Mental health targets

The mental health targets are:

(1) To improve significantly the health and social functioning of mentally ill people.

(2)   To reduce the overall suicide rate by at least 15% by the year 2000
      (from 11.1 per 100,000 population to no more than 9.4).
(3)   To reduce the suicide rate of severely mentally ill people by at least
      33% by the year 2000 (from the estimate of 15% in 1990 to no more
      than 10%).

These targets are frequently criticized as inadequate. The White Paper
itself acknowledges the paucity of the data on which they are based. The
importance they have is not the targets themselves but the practical
changes which will be needed in service delivery in order that they can
be met.

Target (1) – to improve significantly the health and social functioning of mentally ill people

This will be mainly the province of those working in the secondary care
and specialist services. It highlights the importance of good social care
as well as medical care for people with mental illness. There is widespread recognition that helping this group enhance their daily living
skills, social interaction and family support can prevent relapse and re-
admission to hospital. Newton (1992) reviews the research evidence and
details a number of practical projects which have tried to address the
problems associated with the care of people with chronic schizophrenia
in the community.

Roberts *et al.* (1992) describe a supported living scheme in Clwyd
which was shown to have reduced re-admission rates in people suffering
the residual effects of major mental illness. The project team included
community psychiatric nurses, social workers and an occupational
therapist.

Chronic mental illness and primary care

Although this is a specialized field, people with major psychotic illness
(and their families and carers) also have GPs, and will therefore come
into contact with practice nurses, health visitors and other community
nurses. A number of points arise from this with regard to health promotion and medical/nursing care.

People with these illnesses are often excluded from health promotion
activities in health centres and surgeries, perhaps because they are
perceived as a nuisance by the practice receptionist who is responsible
for inviting patients to attend clinic sessions. A great deal of unconscious
selection of patients for health promotion clinics goes on, by staff as well
as patients. This could be one reason why such clinics are sometimes

accused of pandering to the 'worried well', though it is worth noting that the person who is worried is not entirely well. In view of the higher death rates from common physical illnesses suffered by those with serious mental disorder, is this selection logical or fair?

A number of strategies have been developed for making health promotion activities accessible to members of ethnic minority communities. Similar attention needs to be paid to the physical health needs of the mentally ill. Admittedly this may not be easy, but ways must be found if preventable ill-health is to be avoided.

Practice nurses with limited psychiatric knowledge are not infrequently asked to give regular injections of anti- psychotic medication to people with chronic schizophrenia. Sometimes these patients lose contact with the specialist services. The six-monthly turnover of junior hospital doctors is often cited as a reason why patients fail to keep outpatient appointments. They are said to dislike the lack of continuity this turnover brings.

Just as often, the practice nurse herself may have no contact with appropriately trained colleagues. This may mean that patients are losing out on the social care which is essential if relapse is to be prevented. Such problems might be thought to be peculiar to inner city areas, but anecdotal evidence suggests they may be more widespread.

Symptom control may also be inadequate if the practice nurse herself is insufficiently skilled in recognizing signs of under- or over-dosing. Various mechanisms exist which could be used to minimize these difficulties. The first is the UKCC Code of Professional Conduct (1992) which states that nurses should 'acknowledge any limitations in (their) knowledge and competence and decline any duties or responsibilities unless able to perform them in a safe and skilled manner'. This is not suggesting that practice nurses, or district nurses, should not give anti-psychotic medication. But it does mean that if they perform this task, they should understand the full implications of the care they are giving. There are clear implications here for an educational role for specialist nurses such as community psychiatric nurses (CPNs).

Second, since April 1991 when the care programme approach (Department of Health, 1990) was introduced, all patients referred to or discharged from specialist psychiatric care should have a written care plan agreed with the patient and his/her carers, and should have a named key worker. Non-specialist community nurses participating in the care of mentally ill people should ensure that they know who the key worker is, and should maintain regular contact.

Essex *et al.* (1990) describe a pilot project which introduced a system of 'shared care' involving a patient-held record card for patients suffering from chronic mental illness. Ironically it seems that those who appreciated the system most were the patients. Professionals involved, with the exception of GPs, were much less enthusiastic, perhaps because of perceived threats to their authority. Schemes such as this can offer a real partnership in care between professionals and their clients, and a real opportunity for enhanced inter-professional working. It is clearly what patients want.

Working across professional boundaries, aiding communication and building bridges is an important area of work being developed by facilitators (Armstrong 1993), many of whom are nurses. Developing collaborative patterns of working such as shared care systems could be the single largest contribution to the achievement of Target (1). The perpetuation of intra- and inter-professional rivalries and jealousies helps no one, least of all vulnerable clients (Jenkins *et al.*, 1992).

Target (2) – to reduce the overall suicide rate

Most people who commit suicide tell someone, usually their doctor, about their intentions beforehand. Most of these people are depressed, but depression is not well recognized. In the light of this, the White Paper considers that there are many missed opportunities for the recognition and treatment of people at risk of suicide. A worrying rise in the suicide rate among young men is noted, though currently unexplained. To prevent suicide, it is first necessary to learn to recognize depression (Solomon & Patch, 1974).

Target (3) – to reduce the suicide rate of severely mentally ill people

This target again focuses on the specialized services and highlights the need for better information about suicide among the mentally ill. Much of what has already been said about Target (1) applies here too.

Mental health and primary care

How the system works

The primary care system in Britain is based on general practice – that is, on a network of family doctors who provide a consultation service to those who perceive themselves to be ill.

But most doctors do not stop there. They also employ practice nurses who provide additional services such as: immunization; health checks for people who are newly registered; well woman clinics offering cervical cytology, breast examination and family planning advice; health promotion clinics, usually addressing heart disease risk factors; disease management clinics, for example for people with asthma, diabetes or hypertension; and annual health checks for people over 75.

In most parts of the country health authority or trust-employed district nurses and health visitors are also attached to and work with general practice staff as part of the primary health care team. There may be other professionals involved such as counsellors, social workers or clinical psychologists, but this is more rare.

The salient point about all of these services is that they are almost entirely concerned with physical care. Mental health needs are rarely acknowledged, and even where they are recognized, meeting them is a haphazard and unsystematic affair. There are widely used protocols for the care and management of people with asthma and diabetes. Few protocols exist for the care of people with depressive illness, though there are indications from ongoing research (Wilkinson, 1992) that their use would have benefits well beyond improved patient care.

Depression and primary care

Depression is by far the commonest mental illness, affecting about one in four of the population at some time in their lives. Over 90% of people with mental illness remain within the primary care sector and are never referred to the specialized services (Goldberg & Huxley, 1980). The majority of these people are likely to be suffering from depression, anxiety or a mixture of the two. It is therefore within the primary care sector that the greatest potential for the early detection and treatment of, and prevention of, these conditions lies (Jenkins, 1992). The scope for mental health education and promotion is also enormous and hardly begun.

Depression is often seen as an understandable reaction to unfavourable life events or circumstances – to bereavement, social isolation or severe physical illness, for instance. Such depression is often termed reactive as distinct from endogenous depression which is considered to arise for no apparent reason. However, Blacker & Clare (1987) suggest that very little depression is really endogenous. Most is linked to social circumstances in some way.

Moreover, those patients whose depression is not recognized have just as many symptoms as those whose depression is recognized and if the GP is made aware of those whom he/she did not recognize, the outcome for the patients will improve. Those who are recognized get better more quickly than those who are not (Jenkins & Shepherd, 1983).

Depression is a serious illness. More than 4000 people commit suicide each year, most of whom are depressed. In addition there are great social consequences in disturbance to personal relationships, inability to work, disruption of the mother/child bond with possible long term consequences to the mental health of the child, and the effects of low self esteem and low motivation on the ability to deal with the problems of day-to-day living (Newton, 1988; Baldwin, 1991; Jenkins, 1992).

Depression and nursing practice

There are three implications for nursing practice: recognition of depression, its treatment and anticipatory care. We will now consider these in turn.

Recognition

In the course of their work community nurses come into contact with a wide variety of people in situations where a doctor may not be present. This may be during health checks, domiciliary visits by a district nurse or health visitor, child health clinics or many other situations. In all these situations there are opportunities to become aware of the client's mental as well as physical health status. It is possible, in the course of a relatively short interview, to identify mental health problems, and to recognize depressive illness. Wilkinson (1989) lists the key features:

- Persistant low mood.
- Sleep disturbance.
- Lack of enjoyment of usual activities.
- Loss of appetite or weight.
- Impaired efficiency.
- Self-reproach and guilt.
- Inability to concentrate and make decisions.
- Distinctive posture and gait.

A simple mental state examination using three questions can provide the necessary clues to the requirement for more detailed assessment:

- How are you feeling in your spirits?
- Have you been worrying a lot?
- How have you been sleeping?

A nurse with appropriate training might be able to follow up these questions (Wilkinson, 1992), but low spirits, excessive worry and sleep disturbance are sufficient reason to alert the GP to the need for a closer look. This implies that nurse and doctor work together, and that the nurse's findings will be taken seriously by medical colleagues. Those who work as part of a team are likely to have a much better appreciation of the contribution each can make to care than those who work in isolation. Team methods of working are also considered to give patients more efficient and more understanding treatment (Pritchard & Pritchard, 1992).

The use of mood questionnaires, when agreed by all members of the team, can enhance the nurse's credibility. Health visitors' use of the Edinburgh post-natal depression scale (Cox *et al.*, 1987) has been shown to be effective both in aiding the recognition of post-natal depression and in monitoring change over time. The Beck depression inventory (France & Robson, 1986) is a self-completion questionnaire designed to assess the severity of depressive illness, which is important when deciding on treatment (see below). This tool can also be used to monitor change.

Whatever kind of tools are used, the important points are:

(1) That the nurse has detailed guidelines by which to work, agreed with her medical and other colleagues; and
(2) That such methods are used with all patients and clients, not just those about whom 'I'm a bit worried'. Being a bit worried means being halfway to recognizing the problem. It is the current failure to recognize so much depression which must be changed,

There may be particular problems in recognizing depression in some ethnic minority groups. Depression seems to be a universal experience, but its manifestations can and do vary both within and across cultures; for instance, some groups may be more likely than others to somatize psychological distress or at least to describe it in terms of bodily symptoms.

Nurses who work in areas where there are one or two dominant racial groups are well-placed to develop an understanding of the health beliefs and experiences of the people with whom they come into contact. This is much more difficult for those in some inner city areas where there may be a vast number of different groups; it is not practical in such circumstances to have a detailed knowledge of every group with whom one might come into contact. A sensitivity to likely cultural differences is possible though, together with a rejection of stereotypes. People are individuals and need to be treated as such, regardless of racial background. It is also necessary to have a detailed knowledge of local agencies who can help, for example advocacy groups, interpreting services and advice centres. Such local knowledge should be the stock-in-trade of all community nurses.

Empathy and imagination are also vital components of culturally sensitive care. How, for instance, would you feel if you had arrived in a foreign country as a refugee, having possibly been tortured and having lost friends and family? There is a high incidence of mental health problems among refugees, and it should not cause surprise (Dobson, 1991).

Treating depression – therapy as prevention

There are a variety of therapeutic options and although detailed discussion of them is outside the scope of this chapter, there are some points which need to be made.

First, treatment can legitimately be seen as secondary prevention, since those who are properly treated are less likely to suffer relapse or become chronically ill. There is no valid reason for subjecting people to a longer experience of depression than is necessary. Second, antidepressants, although effective in relieving symptoms and non-addictive, will not cure underlying social difficulties. For this reason, a combination of therapies may be most effective.

Antidepressants

There are a wide variety of antidepressants available, from the older tricyclic antidepressants such as amitriptyline to the latest so-called 5-HT drugs like fluoxetine. The tricyclics are tried and tested and known to be effective in moderate to severe depression, but they have considerable side-effects and can be very dangerous if taken in overdose. The newer drugs are said to be equally effective in relieving symptoms, but have fewer side-effects and are much less toxic (Baldwin, 1991). Some GPs consider them to be better suited to primary care use than the tricyclics.

Poor compliance with antidepressants is often cited as a reason for not prescribing them. In the public mind they are frequently confused with the dependence-causing benzodiazepines to which they are not related. If antidepressants are to be effective, they need to be given in a large enough dose for several months. Nor will the therapeutic effect be immediate. It will usually take two to three weeks before the patients will feel benefit, and side-effects are likely to be troublesome in this early period.

It is a waste of time and money to prescribe drugs that are not used. Therefore patients need to be offered close support, particularly during the early stages of treatment. Nurses are well-placed to be able to provide this support. The nurse depression study, an on-going project recently described by Wilkinson (1992), has devised a method by which the care of depressed people can be effectively shared by GP and practice nurse. The monitoring of people taking antidepressants forms part of this study.

Counselling

Counselling is very popular. In surveys of public opinion (Corney, 1992), people often indicate a preference for counselling over drug therapy, as a treatment for depression. Many nurses (and doctors) consider that they are well able to 'counsel' their patients, although firm distinction must be made between counselling and advice-giving, and between the use of core counselling skills such as listening, reflecting and empathy and the counselling provided by trained counsellors.

It is difficult for the nurse, who may have been consulted for a specific medical or nursing task or for advice, to provide more than limited counselling. The doctor/patient relationship is also fundamentally different from that which characterizes client and counsellor. For these and other reasons, more and more counsellors are now being employed in primary health care settings. As well as providing an extra therapeutic dimension to the services provided by the practice, the presence of a psychologically aware person in the team can both enhance the whole team's knowledge and understanding of these issues and help them handle their own anxieties and stress more appropriately.

While it has been demonstrated that counselling is effective in helping some groups of people, for instance women with chronic marital difficulties, Corney (1992) points out that there have not yet been very many evaluative studies. The study by Holden *et al.*, (1989) which looked at the effectiveness of health visitor intervention in post-natal depression is a notable exception. However, there are indications that counselling may actually be harmful to some people. It is not a panacea (Sheldon, 1992).

Other psychological interventions

Cognitive therapy is being increasingly seen as a useful method of helping depressed people. It may be used by a clinical psychologist, counsellor or psychotherapist. The principles involve helping people to recognize the negative thinking which is often a feature of depression, and counter it by examining alternative thought patterns. A typical 'negative' interpretation of an everyday event might be 'my friend didn't phone last night because she doesn't like me any more'. The therapist can help the patient understand that there may be a large number of other ways of seeing this event, most of which would be much more positive (Wilkinson, 1989; France & Robson, 1986).

Behavioural therapy encompasses techniques used by psychologists to change unhelpful behaviour in people who have anxiety or phobic disorders. An example would be agoraphobia – fear of public places – in which a series of graded exercises can help the client deal with the fear in more constructive ways.

In practice, the techniques used by counsellors, psychotherapists and psychologists show considerable overlap. It is possible that the acquisition of some basic psychological skills by nurses could help the care of mildly depressed people, and obviate the need for referral outside the practice setting. An alternative strategy, where there is no practice counsellor, is for the team to build relationships with a trusted group of local therapists, private and voluntary as well as from secondary care.

It is unrealistic to suppose that the primary health care team will be able to provide care for their depressed patients by referral to the local community psychiatric nurses (CPNs) (Jenkins, 1992). There are simply too many patients and too few CPNs. There is, though, a role for the CPNs in educating and supporting their primary care colleagues. Referral to hospital will still be essential in certain instances, especially serious suicide risk and non-response to treatment.

Self-help

There is much that the depressed person can do to help themselves, though in the early stages of treatment a good deal of support will be necessary. The Royal College of Psychiatrists publishes an excellent leaflet with ideas, copies of which can be obtained from the address at the end of this chapter. There is also a useful section in Wilkinson (1989).

Anticipatory care

In theory at least, it ought to be possible to recognize people who are vulnerable to becoming depressed, and to provide preventive support (RCGP, 1981; Newton, 1988). We know what the risk factors are. They centre around difficulties related to partner, family, employment, physical health, housing and money. We also know that certain groups are particularly vulnerable: the elderly, bereaved, socially isolated, physically disabled, and those with chronic, painful or life-threatening conditions (Jenkins, 1992). Recent experience using a semi-structured interview designed to identify and offer support to vulnerable people in general practice suggests that there is potential for further developments along these lines (Armstrong, unpublished).

Contrary to opinions expressed by some doctors, nurses have found that it is possible to ask people quite detailed questions about their worries and social situation. Most people do not regard this as an intrusion if the interview is sensitively handled. In fact, many express appreciation at being given the time to talk. The important thing is that the interview has a purpose and takes a practical, problem-solving approach to helping people identify those difficulties that are causing 'stress', that it provides information about sources of help which are available locally, sets goals for action and provides encouragement for people to tackle their difficulties in a step-by-step, systematic way.

The nurse is emphatically not there to solve her patients' problems herself. She must also accept that the patient has a choice. Patients may not always choose the same option as the nurse, but the patient's choice must be respected. Implicit is that the nurse will have a detailed knowledge of local agencies – social services, self-help groups and other voluntary groups, advice centres etc. Practice nurses often lack this knowledge. Health visitors and district nurses usually have it in abundance, another argument for close co-operation.

Problem-solving techniques can also usefully be used with people who are already depressed. The skills of social workers in this area should not be overlooked. A number of schemes involving attachment of social workers to primary health care teams have been evaluated. A recent report by Ruddy (1992) highlights some of the benefits, especially in terms of a more comprehensive service for patients.

Mental health and hospital nursing

This chapter has so far focused on mental health in primary care settings. Much of what has been said is also relevant to nurses in general hospital wards, but there are particular areas worthy of note.

There is widespread recognition of the needs of people who have been involved in major accidents for counselling and support. The link between bereavement and depression is also well-known, and it is possible for people who lose a relative in hospital to be offered some support immediately. But links between hospital and the outside community may be at best only tenuous, and support begun with the worthiest intentions may founder when connections with the hospital are severed.

This lack of co-ordination between hospital and outside also has implications for the care of people with life-threatening illness – an important at-risk group for depressive illness. Information is shared between hospital and primary care team mainly through formal referral letters and reports. This formality can lead to delay, and people may be in danger of being left isolated for long periods following discharge. It might also be that in-patients are denied potentially valuable help because hospital staff do not know of external factors increasing vulnerability. There could be clear benefits for patients if hospital and general practice nurses developed ways of promoting more continuous patterns of care. This would be particularly important for patients who are not referred to district nurses, but return to the care of their GP.

Self-care

Nurses are brought up to be able to cope. In hospital they deal not only with a rapid through-put of patients but also with the aftermath of major disasters, with highly dependent patients, and with death. In primary health care the picture is of increasing demands both from patients and clients, and from managers and administrators, often with minimal acknowledgement of the stress involved. Practice nurses in particular can be isolated from their peers and have limited access to educational opportunities.

Counselling services for hospital nurses do exist but there may be a reluctance to use them, perhaps because of long-held cultural attitudes within the profession. Seeking help may be seen as an admission of weakness, and there may be unspoken fears that such behaviour could mean career 'black marks'. In general practice settings it is rare for any such service to exist at all. Yet nurses who do not recognize their own needs are unlikely to be able to meet fully those of their patients. In addition, their own family relationships may suffer.

Kellet (1991) points out that nurses with high sources of support and higher levels of satisfaction with their support, report less burnout than others, regardless of levels of work stress. Bond (1991), in the same *Nursing Standard* supplement, gives practical help in organizing support groups. Such nurse-organized groups may prove more acceptable to clinically based members of the profession than counselling services provided by management, which may be viewed with suspicion. But whatever form support takes, the important thing is that it is easily accessible and acceptable.

Counsellors are expected to have on-going supervision from another counsellor (which is actually more like personal therapy) throughout their professional lives (Irving, 1992). Nursing is at least as demanding and must develop a similar acceptance that support is an integral part of professional practice.

Conclusion

At the beginning of this chapter mental health was acknowledged to be an idea which is by no means universally accepted. It is seen, however, to wide practical implications. These have been given expression, to some extent at least, in *Health of the Nation* (HMSO, 1992), which is a welcome attempt to include a mental dimension in the concept of health, and to set some targets for improvement in the mental health of people in England.

There is a long way to go before health care is truly holistic but the field is wide open for innovation and research. Some ideas have been given, but there remain many challenges. Meeting them will mean confronting entrenched attitudes and time-hallowed practices – but nothing is immutable. Nursing could take a lead in developing psychologically-aware health care. Alternatively we could wait for others to show us the way – their way.

We need tools to help us – guidelines, protocols, literature and other sources of information for patients and clients – and we need ways of auditing the care we are giving. Again, we can develop our own or wait for others to do it for us.

These are some of the choices we have. What we do not have is a choice about whether we should take a positive attitude to mental health. The need is enormous, and it will not go away.

Sources of information

Help is at Hand – a series of five leaflets and accompanying posters on depression; anxiety and phobias; anorexia and bulimia; bereavement; and surviving adolescence. Available from: Royal College of Psychiatrists, 17 Belgrave Square, London SW1X 8PG. Each of these leaflets contains further useful addresses.

MIND and the Mental Health Foundation produce series of leaflets on a variety of mental health issues and problems. Write for a publications list to the addresses below, or contact your local MIND branch (see telephone directory or public library). Addresses: MIND, 22 Harley Street, London W1N 2ED. Mental Health Foundation, 8 Hallam Street, London W1N 6DH.

References

Armstrong, E. (1992) On the front line. *Nursing Times*, **88** (23) 31–2.
Armstrong, E. (1993) Mental Health – a primary care perspective. In press, Keele University.

Baldwin, D. (1991) Recognition and treatment of depressed patients. *Practice Nurse*, May, 38–42.

Blacker, C.V.R. & Clare, A. (1987) Depressive disorder in primary care. *British Journal of Psychiatry*, **150**, 737–51.

Bond, M. (1991) Setting up groups – a practical guide. *Nursing Standard* **5** (48) 47–51.

Corney, R. (1992) The effectiveness of counselling in general practice. *International Review of Psychiatry*, **4** (3/4) 331–7.

Cox, J.L., Holden, J.M. & Sagovsky, R. (1987) Detection of Postnatal Depression, Development of the 10-item Edinburgh Postnatal Depression Scale. *British Journal of Psychiatry*, **150**, 782–6.

Department of Health (1990) The care programme approach for people with a mental illness referred to the specialist psychiatric services. *Joint Health and Social Services Circular HC(90)23/LASSL(90)11*.

Dobson, S.M. (1991) *Transcultural Nursing*. Scutari Press, London.

Essex, B. Doig, R. & Renshaw, J. (1990) Pilot study of records of shared care for people with mental illnesses. *Brit. Med. J.* 300, 1442–6.

Ewles, L. & Simnett, I. (1985) *Promoting Health*. John Wiley and Sons Ltd, London.

France, R. & Robson, M. (1986) *Behaviour Therapy in Primary Care*, Croom Helm, London.

Goldberg, D. & Huxley, P. (1980) *Mental Illness in the Community: the Pathway to Psychiatric Care*. Tavistock Publications, London.

HMSO (1992) *The Health of the Nation – A Strategy for Health in England*. Her Majesty's Stationery Office, London.

Holden, J.M., Sagovsky, R. & Cox, J.L. (1989) Counselling in a general practice setting: controlled study of health visitor intervention in treatment of postnatal depression. *British Medical Journal*, **298**, 223–6.

Irving, J. (1992) *The Practice Counsellor in Counselling in General Practice*. (Ed. M. Sheldon). Royal College of General Practitioners, London.

Jenkins, R. (1992) Developments in the primary care of mental illness – a forward look. *International Review of Psychiatry*, **4** (3/4) 237–42.

Jenkins, R. & Shepherd, M. (1983) Mental Illness and General Practice in *Mental Illness: Changes and Trends* (Ed. P. Bean). John Wiley and Sons Ltd, London.

Jenkins, R., Field, V. & Young, R (Eds) (1992) *The Primary Care of Schizophrenia*. Her Majesty's Stationery Office, London.

Kellet, J. (1991) *Caring about each other, Nursing Standard* **5** (48) 46.

Newton, J. (1988) Preventing Mental Illness. Routledge, London.

Newton, J. (1992) *Preventing Mental Illness in Practice*. Routledge, London.

Pritchard, P. & Pritchard, J. (1992) *Developing Teamwork in Primary Care – a Practical Workbook*. Oxford Medical Publications, Oxford.

RCGP (1981) Prevention of Psychiatric Disorders in General Practice. *Report from General Practice 20*. Royal College of General Practitioners, London.

Roberts, M., Barr, W. & Roberts, R. (1992) The home team. *Nursing Times*, **88** (32) 30–32.

Ruddy, B. (1992) Brief encounters. *Health Service Journal*, 17 September, 22–4.

Sheldon, M. (Ed.) (1992) *Counselling in General Practice*. Royal College of General Practitioners, London.

Solomon, P. & Patch, V. (1974) *Handbook of Psychiatry* (3rd Edn). Lange Medical Press, California.

UKCC (1992) *Code of Professional Conduct*. UKCC, London.

Wilkinson, D.G. (1989) *Depression: Recognition and Treatment in General Practice*. Radcliffe Medical Press, Oxford.

Wilkinson, G. (1992) The role of the practice nurse in the recognition of depression. *International Review of Psychiatry*. 4, 311–316.

Chapter 8
Promoting Health for People with Learning Disabilities

Introduction

This chapter will consider both the general and specific needs of people with learning disabilities and will identify the key issues that affect their everyday lives. Emphasis will be placed on the similarities in the lives of this client group with other members of the community. Community development and acceptance, prevention of additional handicaps (and reduction of current ones) and the facilitation of a learning environment will form the core of this chapter. A range of key objectives will be explored, including:

- The ethical/moral aspect of promoting health for people who are unable to make informed choices.
- The provision of advocacy and representation rights for people.
- Self reliance and determination in health and social care.

The framework will be based on the principles of ordinary living or 'normalization'. The work of John O'Brien will be cited as a potential framework for the provision of a health education strategy.

Strategies for maximizing health gain and social awareness will be central themes throughout the chapter; inter-professional teamwork and shared care with clients and informal carers will be emphasized.

Specific issues relating to health promotion for this client group include:

- Personal hygiene and self-help skills.
- Body awareness and emergent sexuality.
- Personal relationships and avoidance of abuse.
- Assertion skills and protection from exploitation.
- Body/health screening and maintenance.
- Avoidance of obesity.
- Self-help skills and mastery of home economics.

- Exercise, physical fitness and use of leisure time.
- Oral hygiene and dental health.
- Mobility, posture and seating for multiple handicap.
- Epilepsy and diabetic management.
- Mental health, to include stress management, anxiety reduction.

Community awareness and development will form the final strand of this chapter, with emphasis placed on new opportunities for integration for people as they leave institutional care.

The nature of learning disabilities

The past few decades have witnessed a number of significant changes in the care of people with a learning disability. They have been influenced by political, social and economic factors and by new demands for responsive care and treatment from informed users of public services and their carers in the community. Perhaps one of the most fundamental and important changes has been a shift in emphasis to introduce a partnership between people with learning disabilities, their families and professionals. This has resulted in the provision of a range of inter-vention strategies which have been carefully co-ordinated within a multi-agency context of care.

The health care needs of people with a learning disability are similar to many other members of the society within which they live. They have similar needs, wants and ambitions; the majority are not ill and all have a basic right to participate in the everyday life of their neighbourhood (Towell & Beardshaw, 1991). Learning disability has over the years been the subject of a number of misconceptions, stereotypes which assume that people with learning disabilities are 'all the same', that 'they can do nothing for themselves' and that 'they are unable to learn new skills or make progress towards independence'.

The titles that have been attributed to this client group (for example, mentally handicapped, subnormal and mentally deficient) reflect in part the different perceptions that the general population and professional carers have had towards people with learning disabilities. For example, negative associations are attributed to terms such as mental sub-normality or handicap. A challenge therefore exists for students of nursing to consider the actual needs of people as individuals, rather than judging them in accordance with subjective stereotypes which may have been produced as the result of negative associations or 'labelling'. This chapter introduces a rather different approach and emphasizes the more positive role that nurses may assume as they work in partnership with people with learning disabilities and their families, to promote valued and healthy lifestyles for service users.

So what is learning disability? We might assume that we all have a learning difficulty of one sort or another (for example, in respect of computer literacy or car maintenance) but we are often able to compensate for these difficulties by demonstrating our abilities in other areas. However, when minor difficulties are compounded by a variety of other needs, society prefers to attribute a label that serves to offer some explanation for the way in which its members behave. The need to categorize does not always receive the support of the people included in the group, and consequently people with learning disabilities will nearly always prefer to be known as individuals rather than as members of a segregated or disadvantaged group.

There is no simple way of explaining or defining learning disability, since it is not restricted to any one clinical entity. It is a euphemism for a collection of conditions, needs, symptoms and problems that are often collected together and described as 'clinical types' or 'syndromes', e.g. Down's Syndrome. Causes may be linked to genetic defects, birth injury or to a variety of causes after birth. In many cases it is not possible to offer a firm diagnosis (Clarke & Clarke, 1985).

The definition of learning disability is also culturally determined. In some societies, referring to those of 'normal' intelligence may include a number of people who would be thought in other societies to lack the functional and social skills required to be identified as core members of a valued social order. In other cases the background of the professional making the diagnosis may influence the initial label apportioned to the individual. Since people who may be described as having a learning disability are not the responsibility of any one professional group, there may be different interpretations depending on the perceived cause of the disability. Doctors, nurses, social workers, psychologists and paramedical staff may all be involved in the diagnosis and definition of each presenting problem and this chapter emphasizes the inter-dependence of these disciplines in assessing the needs of people with learning disabilities and planning how to meet them.

People with learning disabilities can learn and can look quite normal, but the majority do lack some degree of social competence. Perhaps the most important thing to acknowledge (McConkey & McCormack, 1983) is that people with learning disabilities have normal feelings; our task is to ensure that opportunities are presented that allow these feelings to be explored and developed appropriately, and to enable people to acquire a range of skills to assist them to function to their maximum ability.

The nature of care provision

The way in which care for people with learning disabilities is currently provided has been informed by the principle of ordinary living or normalization (Wolfensberger, 1972). The characteristics of ordinary living underpin this approach, which aims to offer a range of choice and opportunities to people with learning disabilities, from which they may be enabled to participate in real life experiences.

Community care has also been accepted as the Government's approach to care provision for this client group and requires the integration and participation of people with learning disabilities within the full range of local housing, leisure and employment opportunities.

The majority of health and social service (local) authorities now confirm that their published definition of community care will be based on a set of general principles which underpin the philosophy and values of their community provision. These should aim to:

- Diminish rather than accentuate distinctions between people with learning disabilities and others [as fellow human beings].
- Ensure that clients share space, activities, leisure, recreation, holidays and interests.
- Encourage professionals to demonstrate appropriate behaviours and attitudes that will promote social acceptance and community integration.

Maintaining valued and integrated lifestyles

If services are to be as fully integrated into local neighbourhoods as possible, staff care practices should emphasize the importance of involving service users in the planning of their lives and should aim to promote the concept of advocacy and partnership to encourage their participation in all decision-making processes.

Essentially most people's lives revolve around their homes, friends, work and families, and the ways in which they choose to spend their time depend on their personal choices and the demands made on their 'free time' by others.

Many carers are also aware of the need to ensure that people engage in leisure pursuits that are integrated with other members of the community. This contrasts with outdated policies that encouraged people to spend a significant part of their lives in segregated activities with people with similar needs. Wherever possible, such activities are integrated and shared with friends and neighbours. Use may be made of the local swimming pool or riding clubs, and visits to the local pub and restaurant to celebrate birthdays or to entertain friends are common features of the range of opportunities offered to clients. As a result carers now find that they are receiving positive feedback from neighbours and members of the community regarding the integration of people with learning disabilities in local neighbourhoods. Through the use of shops, cafés and public houses a high profile in the local community may be maintained.

This concept of 'building community' is an essential part of health promotion and in order to maintain positive and healthy lifestyles people with learning disabilities may, on occasions, be exposed to risks (compared to the relative security of a controlled lifestyle in the long-stay hospital where many lived in the past).

Taking risks has formed a central part of the debate and it should be acknowledged that an environment which allows an appropriate degree of personal choice and privacy can never be risk-free. From my experience it appears that staff considered this one of the most difficult challenges to accept. Life in hospital offered protection from 'risks', and opportunities were restricted to avoid accusations being made against staff. In many services 'risk taking' policies have been written, to assist staff in calculating the risks that naturally appear to accompany life in the community. Examples of some of the principal risks are:

- Pregnancy.
- Bullying by the 'caring' community.
- Getting lost.
- Accidents when people are encouraged to acquire new skills, e.g. crossing the road.

Work practices will also be determined by the extent to which staff offer opportunities to service users to have certain rights.

People's rights

Choice

People must be offered the opportunity to receive individually tailored services to meet their needs, based on the principle of providing real choices, e.g. where to live, work or where to go on holiday. The right to choose also implies the right to refuse to accept the offer of some or all of the facilities on offer. The right to choose to smoke or to drink is also the responsibility of the individual, but in the case of a person with a significant degree of learning disability the concept of 'informed choice' becomes important.

Informed choice requires that information is presented to individuals in a format and language that can be easily understood. For people with learning disabilities this may require the design of information packages based on personal communication styles. Such approaches may include the use of non-verbal communication systems and the use of visual materials as teaching aids to enhance comprehension.

Occasionally dilemmas may occur when individuals choose to become involved in an activity that is regarded by carers and professionals to involve an unacceptable degree of risk. In such cases it is recommended that independent representation should be made available to clients in order to present an objective opinion. Final decisions should be taken by a multi-disciplinary team, chaired by an impartial person, which considers the individual's request by analysing any potential risks (and legal sanctions) that might result from its implementation.

Dignity and respect

Nurses should also aim to present a positive image for their clients by ensuring that clients present themselves in an appropriate manner to the general public. Staff must make efforts to signal to members of the general public the respect and dignity that they give their clients, so as to encourage the transfer of a valued image to the community. Consequently enhancing personal hygiene and providing opportunities for persons to develop a positive self-image are key components of this right.

A home of their own

Services must aspire towards the offer of a tenancy agreement to their clients. Homes should be selected in partnership with staff and residents and should be in ordinary dwellings, in ordinary streets, as close to the resident's family home as possible. People should also have the right to a room of their own and to have their privacy respected. In association with this is the opportunity to acquire self-help skills to cook their own meals, to budget accordingly and to call for essential services such as the local doctor or fire brigade in the event of an emergency. All of these (often taken for granted) needs may present health educators with major challenges.

A meaningful occupation

A range of opportunities for daily occupation and leisure can be found in many services. Some people are engaged in paid employment (Shearer, 1986), some participate in voluntary activities – thus serving the local community – and others still attend more traditional day centres. Wherever possible people are now being offered choice from a range of available opportunities.

The principle of integration within ordinary workplaces and colleges of further education is not without its problems, however. Educational programmes may be required for both the 'host' workforce and the person with a learning disability, to reduce or ameliorate negative stereotypes or images associated with perceptions of disability. For example, it is commonplace among some members of the public to assume that people with learning disabilities are unhygienic in respect of food handling, or that they have a greater risk of spreading infection from viral conditions such as hepatitis (a common fear held by dentists and others). Engaging in community education and awareness programmes is therefore an essential component of health education, to facilitate the integration of this client group.

Personal and sexual relationships

The right to form personal and interpersonal relationships is fundamental, but is often not recognized for this client group. Images of deviancy and asexuality are often attributed, in a stereotypical framework. HIV and promiscuity are also secondary considerations associated with this emotive subject, which in turn may be further compounded by religious beliefs and the perception of some parents that their child/adult is enveloped within the concept of 'eternal childhood'.

Of course to the informed this presents a major challenge and may suggest that in the absence of relevantly designed programmes to raise awareness of risks and responsibilities, people with learning disabilities may fall victim to abuse and/or exploitation. Many health and local authorities are now acknowledging the right of people to receive counselling and support. Some degree of privacy must be afforded for clients to develop personal friendships, and practical assistance and counselling should be available to help people form and maintain relationships of their choice. Safeguards will also be necessary to avoid unwanted pregnancy and health related risks.

Independence

The right to self-assertion and direction is a requirement in all services. Professionals should encourage people to participate in all decisions affecting their lives and must provide assistance to enable clients to become more autonomous in their everyday lives.

Advocacy and representation

Services are also encouraging and providing opportunities for people to have a right to speak, and to have their point of view taken seriously (see Table 8.1). Activities that engage clients as active partners must be evident at all levels of the service from planning decisions to specific domestic decisions about daily life, work or leisure.

Many services now recognize the possibility of conflicts occurring between the expressed wishes of service users, their families and their

Table 8.1 Involving people with learning disabilities, their families and friends. (From Towell, D. & Beardshaw, V. (1991) *Enabling Community Integration – the role of public authorities in promoting ordinary life for people with learning disabilities in the 1990s*, King's Fund, London.)

Level	Forms of involvement	Positive agency responses
Strategic	Collective advocacy. Encouraging public support; political lobbying; building coalitions; representation in planning; promoting mutual aid; using the law.	Developing partnership. Participation in policy making and planning. Funding voluntary organizations for mutual aid and advocacy. Actively seeking consumer views. Providing information and public education.
Local and service element	Local collective advocacy. Encouraging access to community resources; representation in service management; reviewing quality; promoting mutual aid; fostering friendship networks.	Developing partnership. Participation in advisory committees and quality review procedures. Support for informed choice by users. Services sensitive to gender, ethnic and other differences.
Individual	Individuals gaining more control over community living. Self advocacy. Citizen advocacy. Circles of support.	Commitment to enabling and empowering among delivery staff. Person-centred assessment and individual planning. Individual contract specifications. Case management.

carers. On such occasions it may be necessary to acquire the services of an independent advocate or representative to provide an objective opinion of the needs of each person. The principle of self-advocacy (or the right for people with learning disabilities to speak for themselves) is a primary aim.

Making mistakes

Rather than adopt a punitive approach when service users make mistakes or exhibit anti-social behaviour, service staff should provide support and encouragement in order to demonstrate appropriate behaviours for clients to learn new ways of dealing with situations. Staff should respond to such situations as learning opportunities for service users and should offer support to each person and encourage them to 'try again'.

Service design

Following the publication and introduction of the National Health Service and Community Care Act (HMSO, 1990) local authorities have assumed responsibility for the planning and co-ordination of services for people with learning disabilities. For the majority, care will be provided in the community and clients will receive their services from generic health and social care practitioners in health centres and social service departments. The needs of many will be similar to the needs of any other member of the population, and the approaches required to provide individualized nursing care and health promotion to meet their specific needs will require minimal, yet sensitive, adaptation.

A small yet significant group of people, however – between four and six per 1000 population in the UK – (Department of Health, 1990), may have additional health care needs in addition to the social needs mentioned above. Such needs may be physical, behavioural, emotional or psychological in both cause and nature, and in most cases specialist nursing care will be required as part of a multi-disciplinary support service. The health context of care usually has a physical or organic origin that demands an intensive and often specialized response from professional staff. This has been confirmed by the National Health Service Management Executive's published guidance (NHS ME, 1992) on the provision of health services for people with learning disabilities. In that circular the Department of Health advises that:

'People with learning disabilities have the same right of access to NHS services as everyone else but they might require assistance to use the services. Special care must be taken to ensure that they are not denied health care because of their disability, and that steps are taken to ensure that any barriers to access are minimized. Purchasing authorities should include in their contracts specific provision for people with learning disabilities to obtain NHS health care services and to ensure, where necessary, that special provision is made where the health care needs of people with learning disabilities cannot be met through the ordinary range of services.'

Thus the NHS must ensure that all its primary and secondary health care services are accessible to this client group and must ensure that where these fail to meet individual needs, specialist services are readily available to 'ensure that specifications for health care include appropriate provision for meeting the needs and promoting the health and well-being of people with learning disabilities' (NHS ME, 1992).

Care management

To date the extent to which relevant services have been received has been largely determined by fitting people into services rather than by designing specific services to meet the needs of individuals. The NHS and Community Care Act (HMSO, 1990) advocates a rather different approach: the care management approach.

Care management places an emphasis on providing individualized services for people and requires that we design systems that are sensitive enough to take account of each person's needs (National Development Team, 1991). The government requires each local authority to have in place by April 1993 an effective, flexible and responsive framework within which individual care needs can be assessed and through which services can be delivered to service users and evaluated.

Care management requires that each person with significant social or health care needs should have access to a named person who will be designated as a care manager. Care managers will usually be social workers, nurses or other community workers and they will be responsible for getting to know each individual client and their family, will 'map' their day-to-day needs and requirements and formulate a clear action or care plan to take account of their needs, wants and ambitions.

The care management system requires that service users and their families are actively engaged in the identification of their needs; it does not necessarily restrict individual choice to the current range of services on offer at the time the assessment is made. Care management is essentially a way of ensuring that individuals are connected to all the services that they require, irrespective of the source. It is a model based on the principle of providing the widest range of choice possible to clients without reliance on any one service agency.

Once the care manager has agreed a package of care to meet the needs of an individual, contracts will be assigned to one or more service providers who may be selected from statutory, voluntary or independent sector agencies. Contracts will identify the exact nature and cost of services to be offered and delivered and will contain clear statements of responsibility and accountability. Each case package will also be costed and paid for from a complex system of allowances which will be co-ordinated by the local authority social service department. Care packages are evaluated against a set of common standards and their effectiveness is judged by the degree to which they meet the actual needs of users (Brandon & Towe, 1989).

For care management to operate successfully it will be necessary for health and social care agencies to work closely together at both the planning stage (where major service decisions and strategic plans are made) and at the point of service delivery. It will also be necessary to demonstrate that multi-agency systems are in place to assess client needs and to measure their effectiveness. Shared training opportunities for nurses and social workers, and joint participation in the design of both care packages and service systems, will in the future become an important feature of provision for people with learning disabilities.

The principles of care management rely on individually designed packages for people, replacing traditional models of fitting people into existing services such as hostels, day services and long-stay hospitals. Care management requires that a range of opportunities are provided to service users based on the principle of integration within normal communities, and it requires that people are given the right to adopt and maintain an ordinary life and have personal relationships and friendships.

With regard to social needs, the nurse should be aware of the norms, values and social pressures that relate to such concepts as social class and cultural and sub-cultural determinants, in respect of their influence on health and well-being. These factors remind practitioners that the delivery of nursing care operates within a framework of politically inspired policies that need to be understood if not challenged. These social policies construct the systems within which care is provided and determine how clients will access the particular skills of nurses; nurses should therefore acquire skills associated with political awareness. Accessibility of clinics, provision and allocation of resources, and the ethics of any intervention, all fall within the political arena of policies that shape the human environment.

Proposed model for promoting health and social well-being

Involving people with learning disabilities in all aspects of their social and health care is essential. In Table 8.1 Towell & Beardshaw (1991) suggest three specific levels as being essential if people with learning disabilities are to be truly involved in determining their futures. Issues relating to advocacy and consumer empowerment are also incorporated into a model provided by O'Brien & Lyle (1987). This approach provides the basic building blocks for the design of a responsive system for care delivery, in what they describe as their accomplishments model. They identify five key concepts that must be achieved if the health and well-being of people with learning disabilities are to be upheld, developed and respected. These may be summarized as:

(1) Choice for individuals.
(2) Opportunities for integration in the community.
(3) Opportunities for active participation as equal members of the community and local neighbourhood.
(4) The ability to form and maintain relationships with others.
(5) The acquisition of competence and skill.

To these may be added the need for continuity in care provision, stability and the enhancement of status and dignity.

Working in partnership with people with learning disability and their families requires not only a shift in attitudes and values but also the introduction of structures and processes within the care management philosophy to ensure that opportunities for health gain and promotion are planned and programmed effectively. Consequently, in any comprehensive care planning system, health promotion must figure as a key and central determinant of well-being for this client group. The strategic intent of the NHS in Wales (Welsh Office, 1992) identifies three specific commitments for people with learning disabilities.

- Health gain-focused, adding years to life and life to years.
- People-centred, valuing people as individuals.
- Resource effective, achieving a cost-effective balance in its use of available resources.

The Welsh Office designed a protocol specifically for people with learning disabilities, and in keeping with government objectives advised that appropriate specialist help from local communities and from health and local authorities should be made readily available when required.

The report summarizes current trends affecting the specialism as follows:

- The presence of learning disability in older age groups is likely to increase for at least the next 30 years owing to increased survival; there is little difference in respect of mortality for this group than for the general population.
- Improved life expectancy will bring attendant medical problems. Older people with learning disabilities are more vulnerable to age-related physical and mental illness and higher levels of physical and sensory impairment.
- There has been a marked reduction in institutionalized care throughout the UK (over a 50% reduction in Wales alone during the past ten years); this has resulted in a major increase in people with learning disabilities expecting to have their health care needs met by community health services.
- Some 80–90% of infants born with HIV infections will become developmentally disabled; within five years HIV is set to become the largest infectious cause of learning disability.

Four main areas of investment in health gain can be distinguished:

(1)   The mainstream health services, including the primary health care team and the local acute hospitals.
(2)   The large specialist hospitals.
(3)   Health services specifically designed to address learning disability, but with an emphasis on supporting people in the community.
(4)   Other forms of support which contribute to health in the wider sense, including housing associations and voluntary bodies.
   Overall goals for health promotion may be summarized as :

- To reduce avoidable premature deaths.
- To reduce preventable morbidity.
- To achieve measurable improvements in health status.
- To support the developments that maintain the health of carers.

Table 8.2 identifies the reported prevalences of medical problems for people with a learning disability and it is suggested that for each of these, specific strategies should be developed to enhance the health status of this client group. These interventions should enhance the health status of clients with the aim of reducing the impact of any presenting handicap. For example, the high prevalence of sensory impairments require investment in surveillance, accurate diagnosis and the supply of aids and

Table 8.2 Reported prevalences of medical problems in people with a learning disability. (From Welsh Office, NHS Directorate (1992) *Source:* Beange, H. & Bauman, A. (1991) Health Care for the Developmentally Disabled. Is It Necessary? In *Key Issues in Mental Retardation Research* (Ed W.I. Fraser), pp 154–62. Health Gain Panel of Review. Routledge, London.)

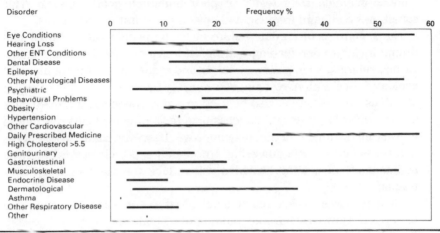

Note: The lines indicate the range of frequencies of the condition identified in a range of studies.

equipment. For others with a propensity to acquire secondary handicaps such as epilepsy and heart/respiratory defects, psychological support and introduction to healthy eating and exercise programmes will be necessary components of a health care regime.

For others there will be a longer term investment need for intensive education so they can acquire enhanced self-help and social skills. This should be accompanied by individually tailored communication programmes which provide opportunities for expressive language. In addition, for those people with multiple presentations which involve a physical disability, preventive treatment and passive exercises might reduce the impact of contractures and skeletal deformities.

Incontinence is another associated problem that can be reduced in the majority of cases, thus providing enhanced status and dignity as well as self-respect. In such cases the combination of behavioural techniques and counselling often produces the desired effect for people with learning disabilities.

Examples of health promotion for people with learning disabilities

While acknowledging the uniqueness of each person as an individual there are a number of instances when specific health promotion programmes may be advocated for use with client groups. For example, although there is not a particular heart defect with Down's syndrome, common cardiac anomalies occur with increased frequency. People with Down's syndrome are also predominantly mouth-breathers (Craft, Bicknell & Hollins, 1985) and they appear to have a reduced capacity to combat infection as a result of poor immunological response. This sometimes results in frequent and episodic respiratory infections.

The symptoms of cardiac failure in young people with Down's syndrome include poor feeding and breathlessness. The signs are tachycardia, enlarged liver, pallor, sweating and cyanosis. Treatment includes avoidance of exertion, rest and occasionally the administration of minor sedatives. Diuretics may also be used to reduce oedema, and medicines such as Digoxin are usually successful in regulating the heart rate and as a result myocardial function may improve. However, many would agree that reassurance and counselling (to clients and their carers) and the maintenance of healthy lifestyles will reduce the likelihood of major trauma.

Much research has been carried out into the causes and presentational patterns of Down's syndrome, but all points conclusively to the need to provide responsive and individual approaches to care provision based on an acknowledgement of the enhanced health risk that may occur from time to time (chest infections, dyspnoea, congestive heart disease), (Cunningham, 1982). In response to these needs, nursing care should be delivered in much the same way as care would be provided for other client groups, but when health risks are identified additional support will be necessary. This rarely intrudes on the pattern of daily living that is to be encouraged for all people with learning disabilities.

In all cases the approach to adopt in respect of health promotion demands that appropriate and sensitive communication is developed with service users, in response to their perceived level of intelligence; the level of intelligence may follow a normal distribution although all have degrees of learning disability. Nurses should also have regard to each person's potential for independence in areas where the individual can perform activities of daily living unaided, such as dressing, feeding, washing and shaving. Through the introduction of sensitive and discrete behavioural strategies, e.g. behaviour modification, new skills may be encouraged and others enhanced towards independence.

Epilepsy affects one person in three but there is no consistent pattern to determine when the condition emerges. Some people develop seizures when they are infants and others not until they reach adult life. Through the use of anti-convulsant medicines it is now possible to provide excellent control for people with epilepsy, without necessarily requiring them to alter or inhibit their lifestyle. The promotion of healthy patterns of living requires that assistance be provided to enable the person concerned to assess the degree of risk that they encounter in their environment, and like others with epilepsy, common sense is required to avoid situations that might be hazardous during a seizure.

Nursing care will also require that individuals and their carers are skilled in first aid (in particular in managing the actual process of the seizure and its after-effects), and the importance of recording seizure pattern and of taking medicines regularly must be emphasized.

The person with cerebral palsy will require the services and support of a team of specialists. Physiotherapy facilitates co-ordinated movement, enhancing the capacity to explore and thus to learn through the manipulation of objects, and to become independent in terms of mobility through exercises and adaptations to the environment or appliances. Speech therapy will be essential in most situations to improve communication skills and to facilitate interpersonal relationships. The combined talents of both professionals may also be witnessed in the formulation of feeding programmes that promote growth. Passive movements under the supervision of a physiotherapist and the active encouragement of movement are essential for the promotion of positive health gain.

Recently much interest has been shown by the profession in the use of a range of alternative therapies such as reflexology, aromatherapy, deep massage and therapeutic touch. For those people who do not appear to respond well to external stimuli through normal channels of communication such as verbal reinforcement, the alternatives of touch, smell and physical contact may be routes for stimulation. Nurses are now engaged in the use of a variety of therapies for people with multiple handicaps, such as cerebral palsy, and also for people who require additional assistance to relax, for example people with hyperactive behaviours.

The remedy may be educational, involving diet (for young persons with metabolic disorders such as Phenylketonuria, a genetic condition resulting in abnormalities in the metabolism of phenylanaline), or involving child development strategies, changes in lifestyle to promote greater use of services, or the general raising of living standards. Nurses have a social and professional responsibility to develop awareness among members of the community of adopting positive health promotion strategies, and they need to be aware of factors affecting the health of the population as well as the specific nursing needs of individuals.

As in all forms of nursing care, prevention is an essential part of any intervention strategy. Prevention may be described as primary, secondary or tertiary. In the learning disability field, prevention refers to the use of a range of measures or processes that aim to minimize the effects that the disability may have on the person's lifestyle and level of independence.

There are, however, a number of instances when prevention may assume more traditional forms, as in the case of primary prevention; for example, the provision of extensive immunization programmes aimed at protecting mothers and their unborn children (e.g. rubella immunization programmes); and the development of awareness among pregnant mothers of the dangers of drinking and smoking. Preconceptual counselling, genetic counselling, good ante-natal care, health education, special diets and improved social conditions are other examples.

Carers who work with people with learning disabilities and their families will also have a major role to play in the prevention of secondary handicaps. Secondary prevention refers to the identification of conditions in susceptible people before they themselves are aware of the problem and it involves interventions aimed at preventing or reducing the effects of the condition on the person's health or lifestyle. Examples include the early diagnosis of phenylketonuria (through the use of universal screening programmes), special diets for people with phenylketonuria, and the use of thyroid supplements for hypothyroidism – a condition that has now virtually disappeared but was in the past a cause of potential learning disability.

Mental handicap nurses most often engage in tasks aimed at limiting the effects of existing disabilities; for example, the use of early intervention programmes to facilitate the development of individuals and to assist the family and other carers to provide a stimulating environment for growth potential. Other examples are social training programmes, skills development strategies, educational provision, interpersonal skills-awareness training, survival skills, habilitation and rehabilitation. Without doubt tertiary prevention is the major arena where nurses have a positive contribution to make to the health of individuals and their families.

Finally, the importance of diet and nutrition must be noted. For some, obesity will be a major factor (as in Prader Willi Syndrome – a metabolic disorder) and in others with profound or multiple handicaps an adequate and balanced diet must be ensured to prevent malnutrition and further cognitive dysfunction. For persons who are dependent on being fed, the latter point is particularly important as evidence suggests that absorption rates in the gut may be reduced, resulting in pressure sores, recurrent infections, reduced sensory awareness and, rarely, death (Mamel, 1989).

Summary and conclusion

Learning disability is not an illness. It is important that people with learning disabilities are not treated as a homogenous group, but as individuals who differ as much from one another as any other group. Their health needs, while being rather more prominent, are similar to those of the rest of the population.

Their strengths and needs result predominantly from their capacity to learn to communicate and to interact with their peers and their environment. As dependency on the long-stay hospitals reduces, in favour of care in the community, it is obvious that the community must respond by developing the capacity to meet the general and specific needs of people with learning disabilities.

Sensitive responses will also be required from their carers, in order to promote self-help groups and local networks of mutual support. The carers' capacity to care and to cope will also be enhanced by the development of trusting partnerships with professionals. One of the key tasks for professionals in the future must be to pass on their skills to informal carers and to the wider community.

The primary role of the NHS in this area in terms of investment in health gain is to create a satisfactory balance between local, accessible, generic services and specialized services. The basic source of health care must be the primary health care team and its emphasis on health promotion (and the prevention of ill health).

This chapter has considered some of these needs within a framework that emphasizes the rights of these individuals to live as integrated members of society and to participate in all aspects of everyday cultural life as far as they are able. The mediators to achieving this goal are clearly carers and professional support staff who must employ imaginative responses, processes and programmes to enhance the health status in terms of demonstrable health gain.

In support of this objective it has been suggested that a care management approach be adopted to identify the actual needs of people and their primary carers. Through the application of John O'Brien's accomplishments model, the values that underpin ordinary living assist professionals in making a reality of community care and enabling people with learning disabilities to achieve some self-determination and self-reliance, reducing the consequences of their disabilities and enhancing their health status.

References

Brandon, D. & Towe, N. (1989) *Free to Choose – An Introduction to Service Brokerage.* Good Impressions Publishing Ltd, London.

Clarke, A.M. & Clarke, A.D. (1985) *Mental Deficiency – the Changing Outlook.* Methuen, London.

Craft, M., Bicknell, J. & Hollins, S. (1985) *Mental Handicap – a Multi-Disciplinary Approach.* Bailliere-Tindall, London.

Cunningham, C. (1982) *Down's Syndrome: a Guide for Parents*. Souvenir Press, London.

Department of Health (1990) *Statistical Bulletin 2/90*. Her Majesty's Stationery Office, London.

HMSO (1990) *National Health Service and Community Care Act*, C.19. Her Majesty's Stationery Office, London.

Mamel, J.J. (1989) Percutaneous Endospic Gastrostomy. *The American Journal of Gastroenterology*, **84** (7) 369–77.

McConkey, R. & McCormack, B. (1983) *Fact Sheets*. St Michael's House Research, Dublin.

National Development Team (1991) *The Andover Case Management Project*. National Development Team, London.

NHS ME (1992) *Health Services for People with Learning Disabilities (Mental Handicap)*. National Health Service Management Executive Health Service Guidelines. HSG(92)42. NHS Management Executive, London.

O'Brien, J. & Lyle, C. (1987) *Framework for Accomplishment*. Responsive Service Systems Associates, Georgia.

Shearer, A. (1986) *Building Community with People with Mental Handicaps, their Families and Friends*. Campaign for People with Mental Handicaps and King Edward's Hospital Fund for London, London.

Towell, D. Beardshaw, V. (1991) *Enabling Community Integration – the role of public authorities in promoting an ordinary life for people with learning disabilities in the 1990s*. King's Fund, London.

Welsh Office (1992) NHS Directorate *Protocol for Investment in Health Gain - Mental Handicap (Learning Disability)*. Welsh Office Planning Forum. Her Majesty's Stationery Office, Cardiff.

Wolfensberger, W. (1972) *The Principles of Normalisation in Human Services*. National Institute on Mental Retardation, Toronto.

Chapter 9
Promoting Effective Drug Taking by Elderly People in the Community

Introduction

The changing demographic profile of Britain, characterized by growing numbers of elderly people living in its community, has given rise in recent years to an increased focus on the needs of this age group. In particular, promoting the health of older people is being seen as a legitimate field of activity for care professionals from a variety of backgrounds (Littlewood, 1989; Whetstone & Reid, 1991).

These changes in societal structure and consequent approaches to care have been accompanied by the so called pharmaceutical revolution (Royal College of Physicians [RCP], 1984), which has not only extended average life expectancy, but also contributed to society significant numbers of 'quality adjusted life years' (Denham, 1990a). Such trends have combined to produce a prima facie link between medicines and the health of the elderly, with the associated implication that where ineffective medicine taking occurs, for whatever reason, the role of the health promoter is to redress this situation. This has given rise to both the appropriation, and a consequent critique, of models of health promotion based loosely on this medically orientated approach.

This chapter will seek to:

- Discuss the extent and consequences of inappropriate/ineffective drug taking by the elderly.
- Identify concerns which need to be addressed by care professionals in seeking models/strategies to promote effective drug taking (including reasons for 'non-compliance' and the related issue of what health means to the elderly).
- Identify, from research findings, approaches which may be advocated as appropriate to this area of health promotion.
- Highlight theoretical and practical limitations of these models and research recommendations, in terms of actual clinical practice.

- Suggest some ways forward for practitioners faced with these challenges.

Medicines for the elderly – use, misuse and limitations

The RCP report *Medication for the Elderly* (1984), while acknowledging the contribution to care of the elderly of modern medicines, also commented that such improvements had been 'bought' at the expense of an accompanying increase in adverse drug reactions (ADRs). This less than optimal use of medicines is ascribed to multiple causes. A disproportionately high level of prescribing for elderly patients by their doctors may lead to unwanted pharmacological interactions. This may be compounded by inadequate initial assessment, leading to inaccurate prescribing and a failure to monitor for therapeutic effect. In addition, altered drug handling in the elderly is often overlooked, resulting in inappropriate dosages being prescribed. Finally, the elderly themselves, when responsible for their own drug taking in the home setting, may not take medicines as instructed and this is an area of legitimate concern for nurses.

The subject of elderly people taking (or failing to take) medicines as prescribed has been the subject of much attention by the health care professions since the 1970s. The medical literature describes this in terms of the extent of 'compliance' exhibited by an individual; i.e. the degree to which behaviour coincides with health advice (Haynes *et al.*, 1979) and is sometimes calculated by the formula:

$$\frac{\text{No. of tablets used since discharge}}{\text{No. of tablets prescribed for period}} \times 100$$

(Smith & Andrews, 1983)

Based on this definition, which, it should be noted, is stated from the professional's rather than the consumer's viewpoint, medical research has found non-compliance to be a major problem among elderly people. Some studies have suggested that over half of patients in this age group fail to comply with medical regimens (Parkin *et al.* 1976, Wandless & Davie, 1977), while one study put the figure at approaching 75% (Macdonald *et al.*, 1977). As a result it has been estimated that some 10% of admissions to geriatric units in the UK are due to ADRs (Williamson & Chopin, 1980), with the further suggestion that this incidence is at least in part influenced by errors of drug taking at home (Wade & Bowling, 1986).

ADRs may well manifest as frank symptoms of physical dysfunction, i.e. obvious illness or ill-health, and, if amenable, may be corrected by the physician. The RCP report (1984) cites the example of the prescription of the drug Atenolol for an elderly patient suffering from angina. In this case concomitant renal failure meant that the drug, being water soluble, was poorly excreted, and accumulated in the body to produce excessive pharmacological effects of bradycardia and faintness. When the Atenolol was stopped, the patient's heart rate and blood pressure rose to acceptable levels.

More often, though, the elderly suffer non-specific symptoms such as dizziness, confusion, 'gone off his feet' or failure to thrive. Such manifestations may be less readily amenable to clinical assessment or medical intervention and may, therefore, be regarded as inevitable sequelae of ageing. However, to the elderly individual they may be equally potent determinants of their view of health and not inevitable at all if caused by a drug being taken to treat something else. Another example from the RCP report is that of diuretics prescribed for presumed congestive cardiac failure in a patient with dependent oedema, and resulting in urinary incontinence. This latter ADR may more significantly lower an individual's quality of life than the original, clinically-diagnosed disorder.

Clearly the link between adherence to medically-prescribed regimens and health is not a simple one. In arguing that health professionals have a role in this area, it must also be emphasized that this role should be founded on a clear understanding of the individual's perspective of his/her own health and its management.

Health, medicine and medicine-taking – the elderly individual's perspective

It has been suggested that failure to take prescribed medicines can be attributed to one or more of three broad causal factors, concerning the doctor, the medication or the patient (Denham, 1990b).

The doctor's responsibility lies in minimizing the potential for ADRs as outlined above, through accurate, appropriate prescribing, supplemented by fully explaining to the patient the nature of the prescription. The characteristics of the medication have been shown in various studies to influence compliance. A complex regime, for instance, may act as a deterrent (Parkin *et al.*, 1976) as may the presence of side effects (Haynes *et al.*, 1979, Norton, 1982). Presentation is also important, since child-resistant containers (CRCs) and bubble and blister packs are particularly difficult to handle (Macdonald & Macdonald, 1982).

Although these factors are useful pointers to decisions relating to drug prescription and administration, they are, in themselves, only relevant when seen within the context of the individual patient's circumstances. For instance, small bottles or CRCs are only a problem when the patient has difficulty with manipulation (in, for instance, the presence of arthritis). Similarly, small print on labels is a hindrance only when eyesight is failing. The fact that these functional difficulties are more common in the elderly is merely an indication for more careful and accurate assessment.

There are additional, though less clear cut, patient-related characteristics which may alert the health care professional to the danger of noncompliance. One of these is general mental functioning, which may be a predictor of poor drug taking behaviour (Macdonald & Macdonald, 1982, Shannon, 1983). Another factor is knowledge and understanding of the illness, although it has been suggested that it is not knowledge *per se* that is important here so much as the use made of this knowledge by the patient in defining the situation (Hogue, 1979). In other words, the patient may be reinforcing a knowledge base ('these water pills are meant to help my breathing') with experience ('they also mean I have to go to the toilet with great frequency which is a nuisance') and coming to an understandable decision based on a cost-benefit calculation ('therefore I will stop taking them'). This type of rationalization has been put forward as a means whereby the patient can exercise self-care behaviour (Given & Given, 1984) and thus non-compliance may be seen as an attempt to retain some control over the disorder (Montbriand & Laing, 1991), rather than defy medical advice.

It must be said that, in this light, the reasons for medically-defined non-compliance may be the result of non-medical, but apparently sensible, decision-making. If antihypertensives make me feel dizzy when I had no symptoms prior to this, why should I continue them? Conversely, if I am feeling better, why should I persist with this course of antibiotics?

The decision to which an elderly person comes, in weighing up the costs and benefits, is likely to reflect his/her perspective on health. While the elderly, like any other age and social grouping, must be considered as individuals in this respect, several studies have suggested that they tend to view health in terms of functional ability on the one hand, and absence of manifest clinical disease on the other (Blaxter, 1990, Whetstone & Reid, 1991). It has also been suggested that elderly people may perceive themselves both as having good health in the face of chronic illness and having bad health without disease (Williams, 1983). In other words, their subjective experiences may be out of line with the medical interpretation of the situation.

These health beliefs may provide a framework within which to formulate an explanation of drug-taking behaviour among the elderly. In order to minimize manifest clinical symptomatology, such as may occur with drug side-effects and ADRs, an elderly person may decide to discontinue usage and become 'disease free'. Similarly, in order to retain functional ability, if the answer to the question 'are these drugs promoting my ability to function efficiently?' is no, the elderly person may discontinue them, even if they are effectively treating some other disorder.

A separate, but related, feature to emerge from studies of the health perspectives of the elderly is that of a strong 'anti-drug culture among this population (Calnan & Williams, 1991). One explanation of this is that taking medication may 'label' a person as being ill by its very nature (Whetstone & Reid, 1991). However, a more practical explanation is that because elderly people want living to be as simple and decision-free as possible, medication-taking is seen as a laborious business and they adopt the view that they are over-medicated (Cargill, 1992). Indeed, it has been suggested that though the elderly appear to be superficially accepting of, and deferent to, the medical profession, medications once dispensed, are often discarded, indicating an undercurrent of low expectations.

These findings are interesting, not least because health promotion theorists themselves have not been slow to criticize medicine. Both Ewles & Simnett (1992) and Seedhouse (1986), for instance, comment on medicine's limitations in terms of producing health, Seedhouse echoing the views of Illich who went as far as describing medicine as an impediment to health because it creates illness and limits autonomy. If creating illness (through drug side effects and ADRs) and limiting autonomy (by expecting patients to comply with medically prescribed regimens) can be shown to still exist, then it behoves health professionals to look for alternative models and strategies to address the issue.

An alternative approach – working together towards health and effective drug taking

The authoritative critiques of medicine, cited above, appear to rest on two premises, both of which need to be taken into consideration in the search for principles to guide the health professional assisting elderly medicine users.

The first premise is that medicine is a contributory, but *insufficient*, means of promoting health. Seedhouse (1986) notes that 'preventing and curing disease and illness is not the whole story of work for health promotion', adding that 'by prescribing drugs intended to alleviate symptoms . . . health workers are digging only shallow foundations'. This would seem to be consistent with the picture outlined above; it has already been suggested that drugs are not seen by many elderly people to be a general panacea, and the alleviation of clinically-defined disease is not always the individual patient's main health aim.

The second premise is that medicine as a professional practice may be an *inappropriate* focus for health promotion (including health promotion for the elderly). Ewles & Simnett (1992) suggest this is because the medical profession takes control of health and illness away from the people, who then lose their ability to cope with sickness and disability. 'Aspects of life,' they write, 'such as ... old age, have been increasingly labelled as medical and the onus of responsibility shifted from the lay public to the medical profession.'

It may be that this medically-orientated approach reflects a sub-conscious, perhaps defensive, stance, adopted by society in general, as well as health professionals in particular. The RCP report (1984), for instance, while adopting a concerned approach to the problems of elderly drug takers, betrays its underlying assumptions and beliefs by such comments as 'nurses should ... assist them [patients] to co-operate in their treatment; and should 'be alert to ... lack of compliance'. Mont-briand and Laing (1991) detect a similar unconscious adherence to traditional thinking in nurses for whom 'a shift from the medical model does not always mean a shift from the biomedical stance on many pro-fessional issues, including compliance'.

All this might suggest that, despite acknowledged inadequacies in established practices, there may be particular difficulty in relating this awareness to health promotion in the areas both of elderly care and of drug-taking. Difficulty notwithstanding, however, alternative philos-ophies of health promotion and nursing research related to elderly drug takers have been put forward in recent years. One such alternative is based on the health belief model, developed by social psychologists in the 1950s, in recognition of the cost-benefit calculation involved in health choices alluded to above. The model seeks to explain the like-lihood of an individual undertaking recommended preventive health actions. This, in turn, depends on the patient's perception of his level of susceptibility to, and the severity of, an illness of potential concern to him, together with the possible benefits on the one hand and barriers on the other, of any health action which might be taken in relation to this (Becker *et al.*, 1979).

Health promotion theories based on this model see the need to enter into this debate with the patient to facilitate informed decision making. Seedhouse (1986), for instance, describes health education in terms of the provision of full information (pros *and* cons), empowering a person to choose autonomously. This emphasis is perhaps not unfamiliar to nurses (particularly community nurses) working within a nursing process framework in formulating a care plan in partnership with a patient. Indeed, it has been applied to drug taking behaviour in the area of cancer care, where side-effects can act as a potent disincentive to adherence (Given & Given, 1984).

In keeping with the shift of focus from health professional to partnership in health decision-making, it has been suggested that compliance should be redefined in terms of 'the behaviour, or set of behaviours that the patient performs at the suggestion of, with the encouragement of, or in joint agreement with, a health care promoter, in order to maintain his/her health status' (Given & Given, 1984). In fact, a number of health professionals (particularly nurses) have commented on the coercive, authoritative connotations of the term compliance (Wade & Bowling, 1986, Webb *et al.*, 1990) which sits uneasily with humanistic health promotion ideals, and Moughton (1982) offered the alternative term 'contracting' to describe the 'therapeutic alliance', which is perhaps a better description of expected client (and professional) behaviour in this area.

Research has indicated that this move towards a philosophy of partnership in health promotion is actually successful. Studies fall broadly into two categories: those based on a straightforward educational approach (mainly initiated by physicians) and those building on this by introducing knowledge-based responsibility through programmes of self-administration (often initiated by nurses).

Patient education strategies include a variety of patient-focused interventions, such as simple, verbal information-giving (Macdonald *et al.*, 1977; Edwards & Pathey, 1984), written reminders (Davidson, 1974; Wandless & Davie, 1977) and the use of a variety of aids (Crome *et al.*, 1980; *Lundin et al.*, 1980). Cargill (1992) has recently suggested that a telephone call to review and reinforce medicine regimens is a useful adjunct to the more conventional methods of education.

Self-administration programmes rest on the hypothesis that practice and familiarity with drug handling and taking while in hospital will lead to more effective and accurate medicine-taking behaviour following discharge. Patients are generally 'counselled', then given responsibility for increasing supplies of their own drugs with (subject to satisfactory performance) gradually reduced supervision. A number of studies have shown encouraging results following such programmes (Roberts, 1978; Baxendale *et al.*, 1978; Hatch & Tapley, 1982; Shannon, 1983). Those that introduced 'controls' into the research methodology have found fewer discrepancies in the self-administration group on follow-up (e.g. Shannon, 1983).

These findings are obviously good news to professionals in the health promotion business. Entering into a dialogue with patients through medication education and practice allows for clarification and explanation to be given to the patient and alerts the professional to problems and misperceptions which may be present. In this way the course of action which will best enhance the individual's perspective of health may be agreed on, whether it is simply adhering to a better understood regime or removing obstacles by advocating changes in, for instance, the presentation, container, timing or preparation.

The partnership approach in practice – some personal observations

It is perhaps something of a truism to say that, while models and theories look ideal on paper, they do not so readily translate into the less-than-ideal reality of practice. In offering this personal, and hopefully constructive, critique of the approach suggested above, we take the view put forward by Easterbrook (1987) with respect to nursing models in general – that they be considered of value only insofar as they inform, guide and develop nursing practice. In other words, any model of health promotion should be used as a launching pad to innovative practice rather than a definitive blueprint into which practice is forced.

There are a number of problems inherent in translating theories and research findings into practice. Theories deal with a theoretical norm which rarely exists in real life. Research trials may be based on empirical reality but sample characteristics and timescales are often limited and fail to match the clinical profile or the problems that exist in the provision of ongoing care and support. The fact that most pieces of research have failed to substantiate whether strategies to improve drug-taking are successful in the long term is a case in point. We would therefore like to play devil's advocate by describing a few case studies drawn from our own clinical experience (in elderly care and district nursing), which may illustrate these problems.

When ideals conflict: professional *v.* client aims

Scenario

Miss L. was a frail but independent lady in her 80s, living alone in a flat up one flight of stairs. She was being visited by the district nurse officially for the dressing of a small leg ulcer on her left leg, but over time a number of other health issues were addressed, such as the provision of a more suitable walking aid which improved her stability on her feet, and the syringing of her ears which resulted in easier communication, once she could hear better.

However, in addition to the 'official' diagnosis of her leg ulcer, Miss L.

developed multipathological symptoms of congestive heart failure (breath-lessness and leg oedema which made management of the leg ulcer difficult), and a gastric ulcer (manifesting mainly as a tiredness due to anaemia). The heart failure was managed by the GP prescribing diuretics, while the gastric ulcer, unfortunately, went undetected for some time, since Miss L. failed to consider the change in nature of her stool worthy of mention.

The scenario that ensued was classic. The diuretics precipitated frequent visits to the toilet, which proved difficult due to both the mobility problems and her tiredness. Miss L.'s medicine choices reflected a view of health characteristic of the elderly, as outlined earlier. She discontinued the diuretics since they interfered with her functional capacity (c.f. Blaxter, 1990) and constituted a 'nuisance value' far more real than the breathlessness which was 'what one would expect at my age'. What she really needed, she said, was the GP to prescribe a 'tonic' to make up for the lack of reserve, or weakness (c.f. Williams, 1983) – the non-specific, generalized manifestation of some pre-existing disorder (bad leg? bad chest?). Finally, the compression bandages applied to increasingly oedematous legs were becoming correspondingly more uncomfortable and the district nurse's attempts to explain the rationale for treatment were met with the rejoinder that 'you're not this side of the bandage!', to which there was no answer.

The situation became something of a stalemate. The GP complied with the request to prescribe a tonic and the district nurse tried very hard to see things from the other side of the bandage, but both could also foresee the likely long term effects of untreated heart failure.

The issue that emerges from this case is that of the extent to which health professionals should impose their values on patients when health concepts are incongruent. Seedhouse (1986) takes the view that a person can actively choose to undermine the aims of health promotion as long as he/she understands what he/she is doing. This would give Miss L. the right to refuse the medication which would prevent deterioration of her heart failure, in the light of her feeling that this presented as the lesser of two evils when compared to the adverse side-effects.

However, the implications are rather broader than this. Montbriand & Laing (1991) quote the maxim that in a free society the patient has the right to make the wrong decision with respect to his/her treatment. This gives rise to two further points: First, it suggests that a 'right' decision actually exists objectively in such matters (presumably that propounded by the 'expert'), and, second, it suggests the values of the liberal tradition that 'the only purpose for which power can be rightfully exercised over any member of a civilised community, against his will, is to prevent harm to others. His own good, either physical or moral, is not sufficient war-rant' (Mill, 1859).

In the case of Miss L., the GP and district nurse may be said to be promoting the 'right' choice. In choosing otherwise Miss L. was certainly acting independently. But the future was likely to be one of increased dependence as she became increasingly ill and frail, with implications for increased attention from not only GP and district nurse, but also the home care worker for social support and the neighbour, who would be called on any time the 'helpline' was triggered. The repercussions of her decision would thus extend beyond the patient herself as an individual, to the extent that promotion of freedom may be questioned as an ideal.

Coping with reluctance: self care *v*. professional care

Scenario

Mrs S., in her 70s, had undergone a cataract extraction and had been discharged from hospital on eye-drops four times daily, with a district nurse referral. District nurses would not normally be expected to visit patients solely to administer medicine and would certainly find it unrealistic to visit four times a day for this purpose. The aim is generally to show the patient how to manage the instillation or, failing this, enlist the help of a friend, relative or neighbour.

Mrs S. was very reluctant to assume the responsibility which an 'empowerment' health promotion model assumes to be essential. Her argument that she could not see to instil the eyedrops was, of course, reasonable enough, but even the acquisition of one of the many gadgets available which positions the bottle and accurately dispenses drops proved unacceptable. At heart she did not want to take on what she considered a professional, skilled role which might have adverse consequences if she made a mistake.

Montbriand & Laing (1991) note that older people tend to exhibit an external orientation when it comes to health care and promotion; even when they do take responsibility it is often only to place it in the hands of another external agent (for instance, a complementary or alternative therapist). Here then is another example of the health beliefs of professional and patient being at odds, the one valuing empowerment and internal locus of control, the other valuing special expertise which only the skilled professional possesses. The question in this scenario is how far should health promoters insist that patients fall in with their beliefs and assume independence (given that they have the ability)?

The accountability dilemma: client empowerment *v*. client safety

Scenario

Following a stroke, Mr A. was discharged home from hospital with both social and health care support. He was prescribed an antihypertensive agent and aspirin (to prohibit platelet aggregation), in an attempt to prevent recurrence, but the district nurse became aware that he was failing to take this medication because of memory and comprehension problems. Her attempts to explain the nature and reasons for the medication had no perceptible effect.

The issue here is not that of a mismatch in health beliefs between professional and patient but rather a conflict *within* the nurse's value system. On the one hand she upheld the empowerment ideal with the aim of patient autonomy and professional withdrawal; on the other, professional accountability could not allow a situation to develop whereby the patient might come to some harm (UKCC, 1992).

Policy issues: professional ideals *v.* practical constraints

This example looks at health promotion within the broader, organizational structure, rather than at the client/professional relationship level, and illustrates how such structural criteria may affect professional care options and strategies.

Scenario

Mrs D. was a hospitalized patient in Health Authority A, due for discharge on a complex drug regime which included reducing steroids. The district nurse's referral letter informed her that the patient would be going home with a dose box to aid compliance. A pre-discharge visit by the district nurse to check (among other things) that the patient was coping with the box revealed that staff had not familiarized her with it on the grounds that self-administration was not permitted according to hospital policy.

In this case Mrs D. had been deprived of potentially beneficial educational and empowering nursing support because of organizational constraints.

Mr E. had been discharged from a hospital in Health Authority B. when a district nursing assessment was requested. It came to light, during the course of this assessment, that the patient was, in fact, unable to read, though it is not clear whether hospital staff had been aware of this. Obviously this meant that he could not interpret the instructions for the medications he had been prescribed and an alternative means of ensuring that medicines were taken correctly was necessary. Following assessment for orientation, memory, dexterity etc., the district nurse decided that, like Mrs D., he would benefit from the use of a dose box. This, however, was difficult to obtain, since neither the hospital pharmacy nor community nursing management were prepared to support its use.

Again, this illustrates the potential for policy and management issues to militate against professional decision-making.

Achieving the balance: the ideal *v.* realism in practice

We should perhaps preface this final discussion by saying that we believe that for the sort of practical, ethical and philosophical problems surrounding health promotion, such as those illustrated above, there is usually no one correct solution. We therefore present the actual outcomes of the four case studies, not as examples of good or bad practice but as areas for further debate within nursing, whose theory and practice base can never be said to be definitive.

For Miss L, events overtook the situation. She unfortunately fell one night, activated her 'helpline' and was admitted to hospital. There her heart failure was controlled and the cause of her anaemia diagnosed and treated, with consequent improvements on her leg ulcer. She 'endured' hospital, but was retrospectively grateful for the improvement in her health (i.e. functional capacity and reserve). This imposition of the medical model, albeit by default, does pose the question of whether this might not be appropriate in cases where to refuse medical intervention may have far ranging, negative consequences. The case for the medical model would, perhaps, be further strengthened where, as in this instance, the patient's own view of health is based, at least partly, on disease/disability criteria.

The same argument may be put forward for the management of Mrs S's problems, were it not the case that there was, in fact, little justification for a high medical/health care profile (as there was with Miss L.). The actual outcome was based on a compromise: Mrs S. agreed to use the eye-drop dispenser herself twice a day, while a nurse would also call twice to do the same. This represented something of a token client-centred approach, which involved client agreement but not the client empowerment dimension.

With Mr A. the 'unilateral' action illustrated in Miss L's case may have been the chosen option, had not he had a daughter who visited daily and could be persuaded to administer his medication. This could likewise be described as an attempt at compromise, but it could also be 'validated' by its approximation to Reutter's (1984) integrated family approach to health, which combines family systems theory with Orem's (1991) self-care framework.

Finally, Mrs D's district nurse worked within 'the system' by persuading hospital staff to dispense medicines from the patient's own dose box at drug round times and letting her handle the box at every opportunity. Mr E.'s district nurse, on the other hand, accepted responsibility for acquiring a dose box for him from an independent pharmacy, seeing it, as he did, as the logical solution to the problem and safer for the patient than traditional dispensers. She accepted accountability for her actions in an area where policy remained unclear, while seeking, as patient advocate, to formalize this arrangement.

What must be emphasized about these glimpses into community nursing practice is that what has been retrospectively analysed in terms of health promotion was actually far less overtly apparent to the practitioners involved. The decision-making in care was based on concepts and values central to nursing – self-care, advocacy, accountability – tempered by the realism which experience brings, and it has been described in these terms. It could easily, however, have been translated (and in some cases has been) into the language of health promotion – client-centred approach, empowerment, political action and the like. These case studies do not, however, fit neatly into particular models of health promotion. Mention has, it is true, been made of medical, educational and client centred approaches, and even aspects of the societal change model could be said to exist in the need to clarify and change health authority policy to facilitate self-administration of medicines and the use of dose box. But most courses of action tended to involve a more eclectic approach which also embraced nursing values.

There is no doubt that the ideal is difficult, if indeed possible, to achieve in nursing practice. There is also little possibility of avoiding conflicts between the different values which nursing and health promotion espouse when they are applied to real situations. Patient advocacy, for instance, will be compromised when it conflicts with medical prescription, and promoting client independence will be difficult when the client does not value this concept or is unable to assume it. Many solutions in reality involve a pragmatism which theories and models alone cannot provide for, though, as Cabell (1992) has suggested, this does not necessarily detract from their value as a basis for practice.

Less open to debate is the assertion that the problems encountered by elderly people taking medicines are unlikely to diminish in the foreseeable future. For community nurses this is an area of legitimate concern, involving a number of complex professional issues We would suggest that health promotion models which espouse the values of nursing can be constructively used as pointers to the way forward.

References

Baxendale, C., Gourlay, M. & Gibson, I.J.M. (1978) A self-medication retraining programme. *British Med. J.* 2, 1278–9.

Becker, M.H., Maiman, L.A. & Kirscht, J.P. (1979) Patient perceptions and compliance: recent studies of the Health Belief Model. In Haynes *et al.*, see below.

Blaxter, M. (1990) *Health and Lifestyles*. Routledge, London.

Cabell, C. (1992) The efficacy of primary nursing as a foundation for patient advocacy. *Nursing Practice*, 5(3), 2–5.

Calnan, M. & Williams, S. (1991) *Images of scientific medicine*. British Sociological Association Medical Sociology Group conference. Centre of Health Studies, Canterbury.

Cargill, J.M. (1992) Medication compliance in elderly people: influencing variables and interventions. *J. of Adv. Nurs.*, 17, 422–26.

Crome, P., Akehurst, M. & Keet, J. (1980) Drug compliance in elderly hospital in-patients. *The Practitioner*, 224, 782–5.

Davidson, J.R. (1974) A trial of self-medication in the elderly. *Nursing Times*, 70(3), 391–2.

Denham, M.J. (1990a) Adverse drug reactions and the elderly, Part I. *Care of the Elderly*, 2(5), 182–3.

Denham, M.J. (1990b) Adverse drug reactions and the elderly, Part II. *Care of the Elderly*, 2(6), 210–20.

Easterbrook, J. (1987) *Elderly Care: Towards Holistic Nursing*. Hodder & Stoughton, London.

Edwards, M. & Pathey, M.S.J. (1984) Drug compliance in the elderly and predicting compliance. *The Practitioner*, 228, 291–300.

Ewles, L. & Simnett, I. (1992) *Promoting health: a practical guide* (2nd ed.) Scutari, Harrow.

Given, B.A. & Given, C.W. (1984) Creating a climate for compliance. *Cancer Nursing*, 7(2), 139–47.

Hatch, A.M. & Tapley, A. (1982) A self-administration system for elderly patients at Highbury Hospital. *Nursing Times*, 78(42), 1773–4.

Haynes, R.B., Taylor, D.W. & Sackett, D.L. (1979) *Compliance in Health Care*. John Hopkins University Press, Baltimore.

Hogue, C.C. (1979) Nursing and compliance. In Haynes *et al.*, see above.

Littlewood, J. (1989) Health problems associated with ageing. *Health Education J.* 48(1), 44–5.

Lundin, D.V., Eros, P.A., Melloh, J. & Sands, J.E. (1980) Education of independent elderly in the responsible use of prescription medication. *Drug Intelligence and Clinical Pharmacy*, 14, 335–42.

Macdonald, E.T. & Mcdonald, J.B. (1982) *Drug treatment in the elderly*. Wiley, Chichester.

Macdonald, E.T., Macdonald, J.B. & Phoenix, M. (1977) Improving drug compliance after hospital discharge. *Brit. Med. J.* 2, 618–21.

Mill, J.S. (1859) On Liberty. In *Three Essays*. (J.S. Mill 1975). Oxford University Press, Oxford.

Montbriand, M.J. & Laing, G.P. (1991) Alternative health care as a control strategy. *J. of Adv. Nurs.* **16**, 325–32.

Moughton, M. (1982) The patient: a partner in the health care process. *Nursing Clinics of North America*, 17, 3.

Norton, J.C. (1982) *Introduction to medical psychology*. The Free Press, New York.

Orem, D.E. (1991) *Nursing: concepts of practice* (4th edn). McGraw Hill, New York.

Parkin, D.M., Henney, C.R., Quirk, J. & Crooks, S.J. (1976) Deviation from prescribed treatment after discharge from hospital. *Brit. Med. J.*, 2, 686–8.

Reutter, L. (1984) Family health assessment – an integrated approach. *J. of Adv. Nurs.* 9, 391–9.

Roberts, R. (1978) Self-medication trial for the elderly. *Nursing Times*, **74**(23), 976–7.

Royal College of Physicians (RCP) (1984) Medication for the elderly. *J. of RCP*, 18, 1.

Seedhouse, D. (1986) *Health: the foundation for achievement*. John Wiley, Chichester.

Shannon, M. (1983) Self-medication in the elderly. *Nursing Mirror*, 157, 15: Clinical forum, 9.

Smith, P. & Andrews, J. (1983) Drug compliance not so bad, knowledge not so good – the elderly after hospital discharge. *Age and Ageing*, **12**(4), 336–42.

UKCC (1992) United Kingdom Central Council for Nursing, Midwifery and Health Visiting. *Code of Professional Conduct* (3rd edn.). UKCC, London.

Wade, B. & Bowling, A. (1986) Appropriate use of drugs by elderly people. *J. of Adv. Nurs.* 11, 47–55.

Wandless, I. & Davie, J.W. (1977) Can drug compliance in the elderly be improved? *Brit. Med. J.*, 1, 379–81.

Webb, C., Addison, C., Holman, H., Saklaki, B. & Wagner, A. (1990) Self-medication for elderly patients. *Nursing Times*, **86**(16), 46–9.

Whetstone, W.R. & Reid, J.C. (1991) Health promotion of older adults: perceived barriers. *J. of Adv. Nurs.* 16, 13433–49.

Williams, R. (1983) Concepts of health: an analysis of lay logic. *Sociology*, **17**(2), 185–205.

Williamson, J. & Chopin, J.M. (1980) Adverse reactions to prescribed drugs in the elderly: a multicentre investigation. *Age and Ageing*, 9, 73–80.

Chapter 10
Food Poisoning as a Case Study of Health Promotion

Introduction

Traditionally infectious diseases have been associated with over-crowding, impoverished living conditions and generally poor health. According to Mckeown (1979) population changes in the 19th century helped to reduce the incidence of conditions such as smallpox and tuberculosis before medical developments in the form of immunization and antibiotics caused them to decline to very low levels. Health professionals and the public confidently believed that infectious diseases had been vanquished, but even a cursory examination of today's newspaper headlines would demonstrate this to be incorrect.

Worldwide, infectious conditions are responsible for about half of all known human diseases in the community, while in hospital nosocomial infections complicate illness and delay the recovery of large numbers of people (Gould, 1991).

Infectious diseases remain a major health problem in the UK for a number of reasons. In the community, previously unknown pathogens are continually appearing, the most prominent example, of course, being HIV. In some cases advances in technology permit identification of previously unknown pathogens such as *Legionella* (Legionnaire's disease). In hospital, advances in medical and nursing care encourage the survival of very sick people who a few years ago would have died. Immunosuppressive drugs, invasive devices and the patient's greatly debilitated condition place such individuals at tremendous risk of infection.

Finally, both in hospital and the community, previously known organisms not recognized before as pathogens are demonstrating a capacity to cause disease, and the number of outbreaks for which they are responsible is increasing.

For example, Listeria monocytogenes was first identified in 1926. It is widespread in soil, but gradually became recognized as pathogenic to a variety of animals (Thomas, 1988). Later, Listeria was acknowledged to cause a range of human diseases, including meningitis, septicaemia and fetal infection which could result in abortion despite lack of maternal symptoms. Textbooks dating from the 1970s report Listeria as transmissible only from animals (zoonotic infection), but by the late 1980s members of the public had been made aware through media reports that it can be transmitted via contaminated food.

A more dramatic example is Campylobacter, not recognized as a pathogen until the early 1980s and now responsible for as much food poisoning in the UK as the notorious Salmonella.

Food poisoning

These examples draw attention to the rapid increase in gastro-intestinal infection reported in the UK since the 1970s. This emotive topic has been seized on avidly by the press and is the cause of concern among health care professionals and the public alike. Individuals of all ages fall victim, although, as with infections generally, the very old and young are usually the most severely affected.

Food poisoning at best results in a mild, self-limiting but unpleasant illness, sufficient to disrupt social activities and require time off work. Hospital admission for the more severely affected is costly (Gopal Rao & Fuller, 1992). Moreover, the source of many outbreaks has been traced to food in hospital, typically affecting older patients (Horan, 1984; Degl'Innocenti *et al.* 1989). Outbreaks have occurred through contamination of enteral feeds (Navajas *et al.* 1992), and among those who should be able to enjoy their food in the normal way, as forcefully shown by the Stanley Royd incident in the mid 1980s when 19 elderly people died as a direct result of food poisoning through poor kitchen hygiene (HMSO, 1986).

This chapter will focus on health promotion in relation to food poisoning and its avoidance, within the framework proposed by Tannahill (1985). This approach is seen to be appropriate here because it encompasses both health education of the individual and the wider issues of environmental and legislative control. Health promotion is taken to represent a realm of health enhancing activities distinct from the service provided by the acute care sector. Most victims of food poisoning do not require high technology care even if admitted to hospital, while the condition itself should be preventable. However, Tannahill's conceptualization of health promotion encompasses not only prevention but also health protection, which he envisages as a descendant of the traditional public measures responsible for safeguarding the community against infectious disease.

Moreover, he recognizes the need for empowerment of the individual so that he or she can more easily participate in making healthful choices. This empowerment is necessary when the public make decisions about food, owing to the hysteria of the press and the evidence described by North (1989) that government bodies have not always had the best interest of the community at heart when investigating and publicizing outbreaks of food poisoning.

In a painstaking analysis of the major outbreaks attributed to Salmonella during 1988, North points out that although the public health laboratory service (PHLS) laid the blame on eggs as the main source of infection, in most cases the origin of the bacteria could not be adequately traced. In those cases where a definite cause could be established, egg products rather than shell eggs were implicated. Here and in a later publication (North & Gorman, 1990) North draws attention to the phenomenon of bacterial contamination of eggs by vertical (internal) transmission. This idea was introduced by veterinary scientists earlier this century. It is argued that Salmonella species which also happen to be responsible for food poisoning are endemic in chickens, present not only in the gut and droppings but in the other internal organs. As eggs develop, bacteria become established in the yolk, which affords an ideal medium for growth.

North challenges this argument by pointing out that there is no real evidence that Salmonella exists symbiotically inside chickens, or that contamination of yolks via the oviduct into the intact egg has ever been verified. He shows that the Salmonella species isolated from laying flocks is not the same as those species reported in conjunction with food poisoning outbreaks and argues that the enclosed yolk, rather than providing an ideal medium for bacteria, smothers them because oxygen supplies are limited.

Instead, according to North, most traceable outbreaks recorded have originated from egg products, particularly in hospitals and commercial premises, and in most cases there is direct evidence that the rules of safe food handling and storage have been contravened, directly resulting in opportunities for contamination. Mayonnaise has been produced in batches and stored at ambient temperature rather than refrigerated, and raw egg has been used as a binding agent in sandwiches. These practices are unsafe because raw egg can easily become contaminated from a kitchen environment harbouring Salmonella, which, as we shall see later, can survive sufficiently well under these circumstances to be transmitted. Subsequent heating would kill the bacteria, although light cooking in custards and ice-creams, when the egg does not curdle, may fail to destroy them.

North & Gorman (1990) accuse the government (PHLS is a branch of the Department of Health) of drawing attention to eggs as a major cause of food poisoning to distract from the very poor levels of kitchen hygiene allowed to persist despite the removal of Crown Immunity which resulted from the Stanley Royd incident, and from government failure to produce more effective legislation concerning food. At present commercial enterprises may ignore stringent food handling precautions because these call for staff training and supervision which are expensive, with costs not directly translatable into profit. To enable consumers to reach informed decisions, North & Gorman recommend that PHLS should publish reports of outbreaks so they are more easily accessible for independent analysis by the scientific community. They also call for the agencies responsible for investigating outbreaks to be private and independent. This would protect them from political and commercial pressures which are currently seen to influence their function.

Health professionals, like their clients, must buy, prepare, and eat food and so, like members of the public, must make sensible choices which may be impeded by lack of easily available information and in some cases by a genuine shortfall of knowledge. Thus empowerment, as envisaged by Tannahill (1985) is throughout this chapter taken to include provision of knowledge to health professionals as well as to those who receive care. Searle (1987) pointed out in relation to HIV that the public commonly turns to health professionals for advice, but there is the possibility of confusion and misunderstanding if the 'experts' are themselves poorly or wrongly informed. His questionnaire study revealed ignorance among large numbers of senior nursing and medical staff, suggesting much room for improvement.

The same situation is likely to exist in relation to safe food storage and handling, as there is evidence that nurses have a poorer grasp of microbiology than of all the other biological sciences (Akinsanya, 1982) and cannot see its relevance to clinical practice (Courtney, 1991).

This chapter therefore seeks to provide information to health professionals as well as to demonstrate how knowledge might be used to encourage health promoting behaviour among clients. The nature of food poisoning is examined in terms which the lay public can appreciate, explaining the conditions necessary for the genesis of gastro-intestinal infection, because an understanding of epidemiology remains at the cornerstone of prevention. Changes in lifestyle are considered, which affect the manner in which food is chosen, stored and prepared and which could influence the development of infection. Attention is then turned to practical measures for control.

Nature of, and necessary conditions for, food poisoning

This section is intended to explode a number of myths. Many, but not all, outbreaks of diarrhoea and vomiting are bacterial in origin, and not all have origins in food. In fact a virus, Rotavirus, is now considered the most important cause of acute gastro-enteritis among infants and young children in the community and can cause a mild infection in adults. Communicable virus disease in the community is generally regarded as spread by air. This is true to some extent of Rotavirus, but there is powerful evidence that the most important means of transmission is by direct contact, particularly via hands. Rotavirus particles have been isolated from the hand-washings of children with diarrhoea (Samandi *et al.*, 1983), while a series of controlled trials in infant day care centres demonstrated a reduction in hand-carriage of gastro-intestinal pathogens, including Rotavirus, with a decrease in diarrhoea once a rigorous programme of hand-washing commenced (Black, Dykes *et al.*, 1981).

Good standards of hygiene in such establishments are therefore vital. When choosing child-care facilities parents need to consider the provision of sinks and toilets. Hand-washing should be promoted routinely before meals. In this respect health professionals provide a poor example: there is evidence that hand-washing in hospital is performed too seldom (Albert & Condie, 1981) even though the hands are recognized as the chief vectors of hospital infection irrespective of the organism responsible (Larson, 1988).

Viruses may also be transmitted via food. The Norwalk virus has been identified in oysters. Oysters feed by filtering particles from seawater and if grown in a polluted environment they concentrate viruses. As they are consumed whole and raw, food poisoning will result.

Food poisoning of bacterial origin falls into two broad categories: intoxications and invasive intestinal disease.

Intoxications

Intoxications are not caused by the presence of actively multiplying bacteria, but by the toxins which they release into food. Classic examples of causative bacteria are *Staphylococcus aureus*, *Clostridium perfringens* and *Bacillus cereus*. These diseases typically follow a short incubation period – about six hours in the case of *Staph. aureus*. They are characterized chiefly by nausea and vomiting; diarrhoea does not always occur. Symptoms subside as the toxins are eliminated from the body. Neither the victim, vomitus or stools are infectious. The most unpleasant factor associated with this type of illness is that it has originated in some other human individual and has been transmitted as a result of poor personal hygiene. Transmission of the bacteria is mainly via hands. Once again the answer lies in strict hygiene wherever food is handled – in shops, factories, restaurants and at home.

Nurses who work in institutional settings are highly likely to encounter food intoxication caused by *Cl. perfringens*. The source is usually meat that has been prepared some time in advance, inadequately chilled, then inadequately reheated before consumption. The bacteria responsible for toxin production survive heat as spores, then are able to undergo multiplication, releasing their poison which is present when the meat is consumed.

Patrons of Chinese take-away establishments are at risk of *Bacillus cereus* intoxication if they eat contaminated rice. *B. cereus* spores survive boiling and germinate into toxin-forming vegetative bacteria when stored at room temperature. Subsequent gentle reheating to produce 'special fried rice' does not destroy the toxins.

Invasive intestinal gastro-enteritis

Invasive food-borne disease occurs when bacteria such as Campylobacter or Salmonella are ingested in contaminated food. Both these bacteria are primarily, but not exclusively, of animal origin. They multiply within the gut, giving rise to systemic, infectious illness characterized by malaise, chills and fever. Symptoms develop more slowly because of the longer incubation period, but the illness may persist longer. Diarrhoea is usually a feature and blood, pus or mucus may appear in the stools.

Circumstances which permit food poisoning

Before food poisoning can occur, the following circumstances must be present, in this order:

(1) The food (or water) has to be contaminated by micro-organisms able to operate as human pathogens.
(2) The food has to be left at a temperature favourable for microbial growth and reproduction. In the case of toxin-producing bacteria, a sufficient amount of toxin must be released. Bacteria causing invasive disease must be present in sufficient numbers to constitute an infective dose. The amount of toxin or size of infective dose that will establish clinical infection varies; for a very virulent strain or species it will be lower, but will be influenced by factors within the potential host. It will take fewer bacteria to produce illness among the very debilitated or immunosuppressed than among those in generally good health.
(3) Time is needed for bacterial multiplication.

Over the years food manufacturers and consumers have employed a number of strategies to disrupt the chain of food poisoning. If there is no opportunity for contamination to occur the food will remain safe. This is the principle behind the canning process, where food is rendered safe before packaging. Cans can be stored at any temperature and the contents will be safe providing the cans are sealed. Clearly those who buy damaged cans at low cost run a risk of food poisoning because the metal could be pierced, introducing contaminants. Fresh products used quickly are safe because there is insufficient time for the bacteria to multiply. This is why food products today are marked with a sell by date.

The incidence of food poisoning, however, is increasing, partly through the increased efficiency of diagnosis and reporting to the public health laboratory services which collate and publish statistics, but also because of social and economic changes within the community. Methods of food production and preparation are changing as lifestyles change in contemporary Britain; manufacturers and suppliers respond to demands for products, while consumers seek from commercial enterprise products they will find good and convenient. These changes are summarized below.

Changing eating habits

People may fall victim to food poisoning through efforts to remain healthy. Canned and frozen foods are being replaced by fresh products, which may no longer be as fresh as desirable when they eventually reach the table, given the tendency of many people to organize a single mammoth shopping expedition once every week or two rather than smaller daily sorties. The problem is compounded by storage at incorrect temperature on supermarket shelves and in the domestic refrigerator. Additives, including salt and vinegar, help prevent bacterial growth, but the trend is towards bland, additive-free, 'healthy' alternatives. Chicken is replacing red meat, but poultry is regarded as one of the main vehicles for Salmonella because of the way birds are reared, slaughtered and processed in poultry farms and factories.

Today families are much less likely to sit down to communal meals. The trend is for everyone to snack individually and the purchase of ready-prepared food has soared. Food prepared outside the home is inevitably produced in bulk and this increases opportunities for food-borne disease. Ready-prepared meals are very likely to be produced by the cook-chill process. This is a method of cooking and reheating food in bulk according to strict DOH guidelines, these being essential to avoid increased risk of bacterial growth (Houang & Hurley, 1991). Cook-chill has been introduced into hospitals, where careful monitoring suggests that strict adherence to guidelines is essential to the well-being of the consumer.

The speed of modern life and the pressures of work outside the home, added to housework and childcare, have encouraged many people to invent their own shortcuts in food preparation. Meals may be cooked in advance and reheated; a pie or curry produced on Sunday when time permits may not be consumed until Monday, Tuesday or later, following a long day at work. Cross-contamination can occur readily in the refrigerator, especially when raw and cooked products have been piled in together hastily. Food that has been stored may be inadequately reheated. A common problem is failure to stir soup or stew, so the contents around the perimeter of the saucepan are exposed to adequate temperature but not the food in the middle.

Although the source of Salmonella in a kitchen may have been poultry, sufficient numbers can survive on the hands after touching food to result in an infective dose to healthy people, even if hands are washed (Pether & Gilbert, 1971). Heavy contamination of surfaces, utensils and clothes by potential pathogens commonly occurs in commercial and domestic premises. Under clean conditions, drying can substantially decrease their numbers (reducing them to below an infective dose), but not on soiled surfaces or cloths where organisms persist in sufficient numbers to represent a food poisoning hazard (Scott & Bloomfield, 1990). This is how egg products probably became contaminated in the incidents documented in the reports scrutinized by North (1989). When the eggs were consumed raw or lightly cooked the bacteria were still viable, resulting in infection.

Previously prepared meals, including those generated by the cook-chill method, are often reheated in microwave ovens. Microwaves lie between the infra-red and radiofrequency portion of the electromagnetic spectrum. When food is placed in an electromagnetic field, heat is generated by oscillation set up in its molecules as electromagnetic migration is induced. Much has been made of 'cold spots' in food reheated or cooked in microwave ovens. These can be overcome by following closely manufacturers' guidelines for use of the machine and the food product, so that the meal is treated at the appropriate temperature for the correct length of time according to the wattage. This can vary. Some smaller, inexpensive models are of low wattage so the process will take longer. When a turntable is not fitted in the machine the food must be turned half way through to ensure thorough heating. Soups, stews and other products with a high fluid content require stirring.

Another major change in lifestyle related to the new affluence is the increasing amount of travel abroad, on business and on holiday (Cossar *et al.* 1990). The speed of air travel means that in many cases the infection is still incubating when the individual reaches the UK, and has yet to produce symptoms. Most food-borne diseases contracted abroad are caused by local strains of *E. coli* to which the individual has yet to develop immunity, but those travelling in rural areas are at risk of typhoid – a water-borne disease caused by *Salmonella typhi*, which still carries a heavy mortality rate among all age groups. Immunization, though possible, is not as effective as once thought.

Environmental changes

In Britain we are protected against the water-borne infections of typhoid and cholera, associated with poor sanitation, apart from imported cases. The British public has not always been so fortunate. Many readers will be familiar with the chronicle of Dr John Snow, who in 1854 linked an outbreak of the then endemic cholera in Broad Street, London to the consumption of water from a particular well. By removing the pump handle to prevent further use of the well, he halted the epidemic in what is widely regarded as the first epidemiological investigation. By the end of the 19th century the critical importance of separating drinking water from sewage had become established so today we have a safe domestic water supply, that is largely taken for granted. Legislation and careful monitoring by the Water Authorities ensure that agreed standards are met, although outbreaks occur from time to time, including some caused by food poisoning bacteria such as Campylobacter.

The situation may change if water metering is introduced on a wide scale, not because maintenance standards will fall but because individuals will begin to monitor their own consumption in an effort to control costs. Anecdotal reports from families in regions where water metering has been introduced on a trial basis suggest that families rapidly begin to recycle water. Some changes are harmless. Showers are taken instead of baths and the washing machine is switched on only when really full. If the clothes are still in a socially acceptable state this is probably of no consequence, but if napkins from young children or clothing soiled by incontinence are left soaking in kitchens or bathrooms a reservoir of bacteria is set up, with full potential for cross infection.

We have already noted the critical importance of handwashing to prevent infection outside as well as within institutions, and the rapid increase in a vast array of infections spread by contact when standards fall. Small children playing together transmit infection by touch, so cross infection may occur between households. If water metering is introduced in all or parts of of the UK, community and school nurses will have a major role to play in educating the public, particularly families with young children, on those economies which can safely be made and those which are questionable. Teachers, caterers and those who run institutions (e.g. nursing homes) would need to be included in health promotion campaigns.

Few people today can remain unaware of the climatic changes said to be occurring, and most will have read of the possible effects of increased heat resulting from high concentrations of 'greenhouse gases' – chiefly carbon dioxide – developing within the atmosphere. We do not yet know whether in this country we will see an increase in tropical infections as global warming progresses; difficulties in interpreting temperature records prevent us establishing whether warming has actually commenced and the speed with which it can be expected, but there is evidence that wildlife, particularly bird life, is changing in Britain, with direct implications for health. There is an increase in the numbers of large birds (magpies and crows) which carry bacteria, including Campylobacter and Salmonella. Heavy contamination of water supplies by droppings may generate outbreaks, as may the practice of leaving milk bottles uncovered on door steps where the birds may contaminate the milk by pecking through the tops. Victims are typically those who pour cold milk directly on to cereal. Members of the same family who use boiled milk have escaped illness in recorded outbreaks.

Opportunities for health promotion

Assuming that health professionals are themselves armed with sufficient knowledge, two avenues are open for health promotion: empowerment of individuals by providing information to enable them to create a safe domestic environment, and a more political approach, calling for high standards of hygiene in shops, factories, restaurants and hospitals. In reality these approaches are inter-linked. If the public can be made sufficiently aware of the hazards of institutional meals and mass-produced food, awareness of hygiene in the home will also be fostered because similar rules apply. Contemporary lifestyles cannot change to eliminate the possibility of food poisoning because in most cases people do not have the freedom to choose. In today's economic climate both partners may need to work to make adequate financial provision, so convenience foods, cook- chill and hasty take-away meals are here to stay, but consumers must use them wisely. Holidays abroad provide opportunities to relax and escape from the stresses of modern life for a brief interlude. Indifferent food hygiene is regrettably among the hazards that travellers face.

The problem posed by food poisoning must be tackled by raising awareness of potential risks in different situations and working together to reduce them. The community nurse visiting her clients in their own home is in a key position to assess the domestic environment and provide advice. Clients may be receptive, particularly if the reason for the visit is the presence of a young baby or pregnant women. Most people are aware of the need for sterility when infant feeds are prepared, realizing that the immune system matures as the child develops. Its gradual deterioration with age is less well appreciated, so visits to the elderly may provide opportunity for health promotion, especially when the purchase of fresh food is complicated through reduced mobility. When children are past infancy or older people are not involved, the manner in which to introduce the topic of food safety becomes more problematic, especially as comments may be construed as criticism and individuals may quite reasonably resent enquiries about what they perceive as standards of cleanliness.

It is here that Tannahill's model is valuable as it incorporates the notion of health promotion as a participative process engaging client and professional in the same quest for health-ful behaviour, rather than a 'top-down' process. After all, both are faced with the same difficulties when making choices about food; both cope with the same facilities or lack of them in the form of reliable food outlets, particularly when they reside in the same neighbourhood; and if the evidence of writers such as North and Gorman is accepted, they share the same propaganda concerning likely sources of food-poisoning. Anxiety about safe food products therefore becomes a shared concern and attempts to improve local services become a joint responsibility, although initially they may be orchestrated by the professional.

Instead of telling people what to do professionals can work in tandem with the lay public. Interest can be generated both at an individual level when people are visited at home and though discussion groups designed to raise awareness in community centres, group practices and gatherings (e.g. antenatal classes). Women use health services more than men, and as women are still in many households responsible for most cooking and shopping, information supplied to women will affect the rest of the family.

Topics which could be broached include choosing where to purchase. Individuals could be encouraged to look for evidence of handwashing facilities in shops and takeaway establishments. Those who handle food directly (e.g. in delicatessens) should preferably not handle money as well. The need for raw and cooked food to be stored separately to avoid cross-contamination should be emphasized, as well as the need for separate knives and chopping boards. If this is necessary on commercial premises, the same rules must apply at home.

Sell by dates are worth discussing. The date on the product is no more than an indication of its shelf life and if possible consumption should not be delayed, particularly if the produced is stored outside a refrigerator (perhaps for part of a day in a warm office if shopping took place in a lunch-break). This can lead naturally into a consideration of safe storage temperatures – a refrigerator should maintain food at no more than 4°C. Householders may be prompted to check their own appliances.

Many will appreciate the need for low temperatures to reduce growth of Salmonella, but will be surprised at the ability of Listeria to survive at lower temperatures. This fact has probably contributed to the increase in reported Listeria outbreaks, with a higher incidence of outbreaks earlier in the year. Salmonella, which thrives in hotter weather, tends to give rise to more cases as the summer progresses. Listeria is chiefly a threat to pregnant women, who need to be aware very early, preferably before conception, of the foods which should be avoided (chilled meat and unpasteurised dairy products) as this problem cannot be eradicated by refrigeration. In restaurants dishes incorporating mayonnaise could be avoided to eliminate hazards from raw egg. If managers of restaurants and shops became aware of direct public pressure affecting sales, they would be obliged to accept the need for high standards and to enforce them. Reputable establishments are pleased to learn about lapses and genuinely welcome opportunities to improve customer services.

Conclusion

This chapter has considered food poisoning as an example of one among many types of infection increasing in modern Britain. Previously associated with poor standards of living, its incidence is now rising relentlessly as a direct consequence of alterations in lifestyle not necessarily linked with poverty. Although many of the suggestions for prevention are uncomplicated and could be considered to fall within the realms of common sense, many people, including health professionals, do not seem fully informed. This chapter, by extending knowledge, is intended to stimulate those in contact with the general public to increase awareness of the hazards of food poisoning and to encourage health promotion through their own activities in the community and those of their clients.

References

Akinsanya, J.A. (1982) *The Life Sciences In Nurse Education.* PhD Thesis, University of London.

Albert, R. & Condie, F. (1981) *Handwashing patterns in medical intensive care units.* New England J. of Med. 304, 1465–6.

Black, R.E., Dykes, A.C., Kern, E.A. and Wells, S.P. (1981) *Handwashing to prevent diarrhoea in day centres.* Amer. J. of Epidemiology, 113, 445–51.

Cossar, J.H., Reid, D. & Fallon, R. (1990) *A cumulative view of studies on travellers – their experience of illness and the implications of these findings.* J. of Infection, 21, 27–42.

Courtney, M. (1991) *A study of the teaching of the biological sciences in nurse education.* J. of Advanced Nursing, 16, 1110–16.

Degl'Innocenti, R., DeSantis, M., Berdondini, I. & Dei, R. (1989) *Outbreak of Clostridium difficile diarrhoea in an orthopaedic ward.* J. of Hospital Infection, 13, 309–14.

Gopal Rao, G. & Fuller, M. (1991) *A review of hospitalised patients with bacterial gastroenteritis.* J. of Hospital Infection, 20, 105–11.

Gould, D. (1991) Nurses' hands as vectors of hospital-acquired infection: a review. J. of Advanced Nursing, 16, 1216–25.

HMSO (1986) *Report of a Public Enquiry into the Outbreak of Salmonella Food Poisoning at Stanley Royd Hospital.* Her Majesty's Stationery Office, London.

Horan, M.A. (1984) *Outbreak of Shigella sonnei dysentry on a geriatric assessment ward.* J. of Hospital Infection, 5, 210–12.

Houang, E. & Hurley, R. (1991) *Isolation of Listeria species from precooked chilled foods.* J. of Hospital Infection, 19, 231–8.

Larson, E. (1988) A causal link between handwashing and risk of infection? Examination of the evidence. *Infection Control and Hospital Epidemiology*, 9, 28–35.

Mckeown, T. (1979) The role of medicine. Blackwell Scientific Publications, Oxford.

Navajas, M., Chacon, D.J., Solvas, J.F.G. and Vargas, R. (1992) Bacterial contamination of enteral feeds as a possible source of nosocomial infection. J. of Hospital Infection, 21, 111–20.

North, R. (1989) Food scares: The role of the Department of Health. In (Eds A. Harrison & J. Gretton) pp 65–77. *Health Care UK – an economic social and policy audit.* Policy Journals, Newbury.

North, N. & Gorman, T. (1990) Chickengate. An Independent Analysis of the Salmonella in Eggs Scare. *Health Unit Paper No. 10.* Institute of Economic Affairs Health and Welfare Unit, London.

Pether, J.V.S. & Gilbert, R.J. (1971) The survival of Salmonella on the fingertips and the transfer of the organisms to food. *J. of Hygiene*, 69, 673–81.

Samandi, A.R., Huq, M.I. & Ahmed, Q.S. (1983) Detection of Rotavirus in handwashings of attendants of children with diarrhoea. *Brit. Med. J.*, 1, 188.

Scott, E. & Bloomfield, S. (1990) The survival and transfer of microbial contamination via cloths, hands and utensils. *J. of Applied Bacteriology*, 68, 271–8.

Searle, E.B. (1987) Knowledge, Attitudes and Behaviour of Health Professionals in Relation to AIDS. *The Lancet*, 1, 26–8.

Tannahill, A. (1985) What is Health Promotion? *Health Educ. J.* **44**(4) 167–8.
Thomas, E. (1988) *Medical Microbiology.* Bailliere- Tindall, London.

Note. Statistics are published quarterly by the Office Of Population Censuses and
Surveys, London.

Chapter 11
Homeless Families – A Health Promotion Challenge

Introduction

This chapter presents the findings of an evaluation of the work of the Health Visitors Homeless Families Unit in Ealing. It includes a detailed analysis of 309 families who were living in hostels or hotels in Ealing in December 1989. The socio-demographic characteristics are compared with the background population, along with a comparison of health indicators and specific problems. Finally, an interpretation of what health promotion work involves with this particular client group is discussed.

To plan a service to meet the needs of homeless families living in hostel or hotel accommodation requires information. The Department of the Environment's statistical returns on homelessness do not request detailed information on such families (Evans & Duncan, 1988) and a recent study has concluded that current data are inadequate for planning services to meet the medical needs of such families (Connelly, et al., 1990). Furthermore, information needs to be collected at local level to enable a sensitive and responsive service to be provided for local needs.

Our understanding of the health needs of homeless families (the needs of the single homeless are not addressed here) has depended on some surveys (Conway et al., 1988; Hayden & Bose, 1991; Drennan & Stearn, 1986; Paterson & Roderick, 1990) and many reports by health workers in the professional journals (Morton, 1990; Bayswater Hotel Homelessness Project, 1987; Boyer, 1986).

Numbers of homeless

In Britain there is legal provision for assistance to homeless people in the Housing (Homeless Persons) Act 1977 (1983), which is incorporated into the Housing Act 1985. That Act places a duty on local authorities to provide permanent accommodation for certain groups of homeless people who are defined as in priority need, including vulnerable people, pregnant women and families with dependent children. Prior to 1977, people had very few legal rights to housing.

In 1970 there were 7500 registered homeless families in Britain, but there has been a dramatic increase since 1982, with the use of hotels as temporary accommodation. In 1978 there were 53 000 and 7% were placed in hotels. By 1989, there were 148,000, 12% of whom were in hotels. (Table 11.1).

Thus at the end of 1989, 40 000 households in Great Britain who had been accepted as homeless were in temporary accommodation, compared with 23 000 at the end of 1986 (Table 11.2). The largest increase has been in the use of short life tenancies. These figures did not include people not accepted by local authorities as in priority need; in 1989 a further 250 000 approached local authorities for assistance and were ineligible. Wide disparities between local authorities existed and acceptancies ranged from 11% to 98%. According to a report by the Audit Commission, 'there has been a steady growth over a long period of time, across all types of authorities, under all types of political control with widely varying housing policy' (Audit Commission, 1989).

Table 11.1 Homeless households in Great Britain found accommodation by local authorities: by priority need category.[1] (Source: Table 8.13 Social Trends 1991, Department of the Environment, Welsh Office, Scottish Office.)

	1986	1988	1989
Priority need category %			
Household with dependent children	65	65	67
Household member pregnant	13	14	13
Household member vulnerable because of:			
Old age	7	7	6
Physical handicap	3	3	3
Mental illness	2	3	2
Other reasons	6	7	7
Homeless in emergency	3	2	2
All categories[2] (= 100%) (thousands)	112.0	123.6	134.3
In addition, number accommodated who were not in priority need (thousands)	10.2	12.6	13.2

[1] Households found accommodation under the *Housing Act 1985* which defines 'priority need'. Data for Wales include some households given advice and assistance only.
[2] Includes actions where priority need category is not known.

Table 11.2 Homeless households (thousands) in Great Britain in temporary accommodation[1,2]: by type of accommodation. (Source: Table 8.16 Social Trends 1991, Department of the Environment, Welsh Office, Scottish Office.)

	1986	1988	1989
Bed and breakfast	9	11	12
Hostels, including women's refugees	5	7	9
Short life tenancies and other accommodation	8	14	20
Total in temporary accommodation	23	32	40

[1] At end of year.
[2] Includes households awaiting outcome of homelessness enquiries.

Cause of escalation in homelessness

The 1980 Housing Act compelled Local Authorities to sell council properties to tenants at 33% discount. In Britain it is estimated that one and a quarter million have since been sold. The 1980 Housing Act also decreed that 75% of the £8 billion of capital receipts which local authorities accumulated from council property sales must be spent repaying debt rather than building or renovating stock. As a result, since 1979, central government has cut public housing investment by 70%. The resulting reduction in the amount of available housing, and the increased numbers, has meant people being placed in temporary accommodation for long periods (LHAC, 1989).

The last London Research Centre survey concluded that the main reason behind the continuing rise in the use of temporary accommodation is the continuing contraction in the supply of public and private rented property, rather than an increase in demand (London Research Centre, 1988).

Reasons for homelessness

Table 11.3 shows the main reason for statutory homelessness in Great Britain. For the years 1981 and 1989 the main cause of homelessness was the fact that relatives and friends were no longer willing or able to accommodate people (42%). The second largest cause was the loss of a private rented dwelling, followed closely by relationship breakdown. In both years, one tenth of families were made homeless as a result of mortgage default or rent arrears.

Table 11.3 Homeless households[1] in Great Britain found accommodation by local authorities: by reason[2] for homelessness, 1981 and 1989. (Source: Table 8.14 Social Trends 1991, Department of the Environment, Welsh Office, Scottish Office.)

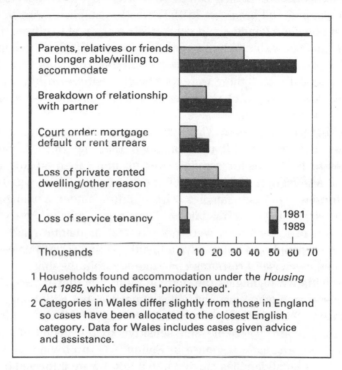

1 Households found accommodation under the *Housing Act 1985,* which defines 'priority need'.
2 Categories in Wales differ slightly from those in England so cases have been allocated to the closest English category. Data for Wales includes cases given advice and assistance.

Homeless families and health in Ealing in 1989

Homelessness in Ealing

The reasons for families becoming homeless in Ealing generally reflected the national picture. In 1988/9 Ealing borough accepted 1192 priority need families out of 5024 applications, in the Homeless Families Unit. Ealing had a total of 9500 families on the waiting list and homelessness was the main route to council housing. By 1987/8 the Ealing homelessness rate was 13.9 per 1000 households, well above the London average of 11 per 1000 households.

By January 1990, Ealing had one of the largest concentrations of homeless families in London. But the proportion placed in hotels had fallen from 82% in 1988 to 38% by 1990 due to the success of the private leasing scheme (as in the rest of London). This was a popular scheme with tenants who spent a few months in hotels rather than the two to three years waiting for a property, they received a property within the borough and were charged 20% of their incomes as an affordable rent with the rest subsidized, partly by housing benefit (Roof, 1989a).

The response of Ealing Health Authority to the rising number of families in bed and breakfast in 1983 was to establish a health visiting post for homeless families, and regular lists were sent to it from the town hall of families with children under five (Boyer, 1986). The number of families passing through the books per annum rose from 27 in 1982 to 1264 by 1990. By 1989 there were four health visitors working 110 hours a week, assisted by a clerk, covering a total caseload of around 300 families at any one time.

The BMA/HVA (Health Visitors Association) report on homeless families and their health recommended that the ratio of homeless families to health visitor should never be more than 50 to 1 (British Medical Association, 1989). By 1990 the average caseload was 141 to 1. So priorities were set: families with children under 5 and pregnant women, screening, referral and welfare rights advice. Every month about 14% of acceptances were for physical or mental handicap and sadly these people did not receive a health visiting service unless it was requested, because of resource constraints within the unit.

This initiative highlights the debate about whether we should have specialist teams who have particular expertise, but which may further marginalize the homeless, or whether we should provide mainstream services that are accessible and sensitive to the needs of homeless people. The pragmatic response in Ealing was to provide an outreach service, so that all families moving into a hotel were informed by health visitors of existing local services, including local authority and voluntary groups, and were encouraged to use them.

It is important to recognize that without social policy changes, the health service has little impact on mitigating the effects of homelessness and poverty on health. Research indicates that although health visitors see poverty as a structural issue, many find it difficult to inform and change people's practice (Popay *et al.* 1986). So what strategies can health workers develop when working with homeless families?

Families living in hotels and hostels suffer the burdens of poor housing, unemployment and the associated higher levels of morbidity and mortality documented by *The Black Report* (Townsend & Davidson, 1982), *The Health Divide* (Whitehead, 1987) and more recently *The Nation's Health* (Smith & Jacobson, 1988). Improving access to health care is only one small factor in improving people's health, but it is within our remit to do it. Other aims include raising awareness of health needs, identifying need and mobilizing resources and providing care and support.

Starting with the premise that these families were already disadvantaged in terms of the effects of poor housing and poverty, and that access to services would probably be in inverse relation to their need (Tudor Hart, 1971), we developed ways of working to challenge these powerful influences on health. Each health visitor approached the task in a different way, depending on the expressed needs of families and the resources in the locality. But all provided flexibility and all worked with the voluntary sector and the local authority.

A model developed by SIGH (Special Interest Group for Homelessness) (Health Visitors Association, 1989) was useful to us in summarizing all the issues (Fig. 11.1).

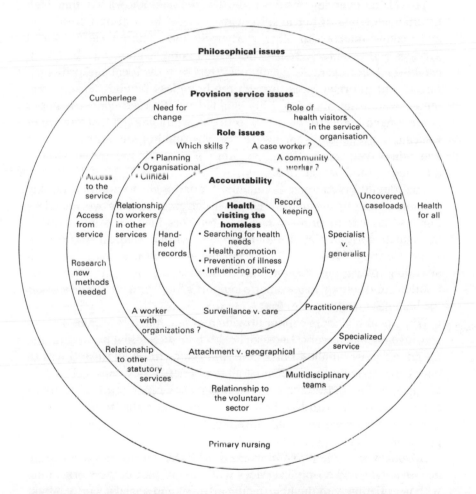

Fig. 11.1 Health visiting the homeless and current issues in nursing. *(Source: Sandall, J., Rowlands, A., Cameron, F., & Sobers, J. Homeless Families and Health in Ealing in 1989. Unpublished report to Ealing Health Authority. Reproduced with permission.)*

Implications for health visiting practice

The Homeless Families Unit covered all hotels and hostels in Ealing which were used by Ealing Borough Homeless Families Unit. We did not cover short life, private leased property or hotels used by the DSS. Because we had great difficulty in requesting previous records and tracking down families when they moved out of hotels, clerical help was invaluable.

The unit was based in a clinic in central Ealing and each health visitor provided a specialist service to each locality, but the unit was also able to provide an overview district wide. The detailed knowledge that each health visitor had of her locality was essential in offering information and making referrals to other workers in the NHS, education, social services and voluntary groups with whom good relationships had been established. For example, liaison occurred with the local authority on a formal and informal basis through the homeless families liaison committee which met monthly. This enabled us to voice concerns about conditions in hotels to the hotels' officers, while being keenly aware of issues of confidentiality. We were also informed of vulnerable families and adults very soon after they were placed by the social worker attached to the borough unit.

The Family Practitioner Committee funded a GP to attend a weekly session at one of the playgroups, in an attempt to improve homeless families' access to primary health care. This had been found to be inadequate in Ealing as in other surveys (British Medical Association 1988; Conway *et al.* 1988). Other health visitor activity included attending playgroup sessions for homeless families in Ealing and Southall, and setting up a women's support group with the social worker for homeless families in Acton.

While health visitors cannot provide a home, much can be done with sensitive outreach work. Because health had such a low priority on the agenda of most families, one of the first issues to be addressed was to check that families were claiming all the benefits they were entitled to. We arranged extra training with the DSS liaison officer and developed a good relationship with her, in that she was either able to give us telephone advice or we were able to refer families with more complicated problems to her.

Advocacy was a key role in working with this group, and negotiating access to GPs and hospital services was a major part of the work, along with negotiating with the housing department and social security. Much information was based on personal knowledge about how to get access to other services of which families were unaware. For example, families on benefit were able to take advantage of sports centres at low cost and some mothers were able to take advantage of courses at the local college that also provided childcare.

A detailed first assessment of a family would often take two hours, particularly if developmental screening was included. The Denver Assessment tool (Frankenburg & Dodds, 1973) was very popular with families and provided a focus for discussion about the developmental needs of children. Growth was also measured on portable electronic scales and a mat and the parents were encouraged to monitor their children's growth using the centile charts in the child health record book. Families were encouraged to attend the GP or local clinic for immunizations as the intention was to enable them to integrate with the standard services and many families already had a GP in Ealing.

The most important part of our work was raising the awareness of other health authority staff to the problems that homeless families have. We were able to develop relations with clinic and hospital staff, so that referrals could be dealt with promptly. Children from these families were often turned away from clinics when they presented for immunizations because the records had been lost. We gave these families their own record books, but this system only worked when all health professionals used the record card. Client-held records were the obvious answer to this problem and have since been implemented.

For some families who were fleeing violence, and for the Somalian refugees, the hotels and hostels provided a haven of support and friendship. But violent partners can easily pursue women into most hotels and although some are for women only, some may contain men discharged from prison who have been convicted of committing violent offences against women (Roof, 1989b). We suspected that many women we met had experienced traumatic childhoods and sexual abuse, but this information was only revealed as trust was built up. Families who were new to the area had many problems settling in when they were rehoused, and again part of our work involved detailed liaison with the new health visitor.

Because we were in a key position to gather and analyse information, this could be used to plan services in a more responsive way and argue for more resources. An evaluation of the unit (Sandall, 1990) monitored caseload profiles in which health and social indicators were compared to small area census data of the surrounding population. The effectiveness of the existing service was monitored and compared to the background population in Ealing, mainly in terms of routine indicators such as immunization and the uptake of developmental screening, but more importantly, as to whether the service was appropriate and had no major gaps.

As a result of this evaluation we identified staff development and

Table 11.4 Results of caseload profile. (Data source: caseload profiles December/ March 1989/90 and Census Digest Ealing Local Authority 1982.)

Social Indicators	Dec. 89
Total caseload of unit	309 families
	%
Head of household of New Commonwealth origin – all	39
Ealing Borough 1981 census	17
Single parent family – all	40
Ealing Borough 1981 Census	17
Head of household unemployed – all	61
Ealing Borough, Jan 1990	5
Refugee families – all	8

training needs and obtained funding to produce an information leaflet for families as they moved into hotels. Also, our knowledge of the impact of homelessness on families was fed into local and national campaigns and SIGH (HVA special interest group for homeless families).

A survey for Ealing Borough in 1987 found 86% of families in bed and breakfast dependent on benefits with only 14% working (Ealing Local Authority, 1989). It is recognized that households in hotels have problems in holding down jobs because of travel and the unsettled way of life.

In the absence of ethnic monitoring it was difficult to estimate the ethnic background of applicants. An analysis by the council suggested Asian households were disproportionately represented in numbers accepted as homeless. Similar findings had been found in other areas: in 1985/6, of households accepted as homeless by the London Borough 30% were black, although black households were only 10% of households in general (London Housing Forum, 1988). We found similar figures although they tended to reflect the population profile of the locality, i.e. 63% of the families living in hotels in Southall were either of Asian or Afro-Caribbean origin.

Immunization uptake among the homeless households was comparable with that for Ealing Health Authority, and higher in some localities, but the low uptake of measles, mumps and rubella immunization (MMR) caused concern. These children had received immunizations on an opportunistic basis as they moved around, hence the 'official' computerized uptake rates for this group were extremely low. There was a

Table 11.5 Health indicators. (Data source: caseload profiles December 1989/March 1990 and Ealing Health Authority.)

Total unit caseload, December 1989	309 families
	%
Infants <2500 g – all	11
Ealing Borough 1988	7
England and Wales 1988 (social class 5)	8
Immunization status	
Completed triple – all	76
Ealing Health Authority 1989	81
MMR – all	55
Ealing Health Authority 1989	50

higher incidence of low birth weight, particularly in women living in bed and breakfast in Southall where 15% of all babies were born under 2500 g. It is important to realize that many families were not homeless at the time they should have had the immunizations and throughout the time of pregnancy. These figures merely show the general trend for families that are highly mobile, compared with those for the health authority in general.

Comparing uptake status of developmental checks with Ealing Health Authority was difficult because of a paucity of data for the health authority in general. A few estimates made in 1988 (Ealing Health Authority, 1990) revealed no dramatic differences between the figures. Nevertheless, many children living in hotels and hostels were missing check-ups because of ignorance of timing of checks by parents, missed appointments, and lack of opportunistic screening by clinics and health visitors. Many children missed appointments in Southall because they are abroad when checks were due, highlighting the need for opportunistic health screening on return.

Homelessness and health

The adverse effects of homelessness on health have been well documented (BMA 1989) (Hayden & Bose 1991). Families in bed and breakfast hotels are susceptible to depression, anxiety and a range of behavioural disorders. Pregnant women are twice as likely to have problems and three times as likely to need hospital admission as other

Table 11.6 Developmental screening.

	%
6 week check – all	68
Ealing Health Authority estimate 1988	80
7 months hearing test – all	50
Ealing Health Authority	*
8 month check – all	53
Ealing Health Authority	*
London bed and breakfast (Conway, 1988)	31
18 month check – all	60
Ealing Health Authority	*
London bed and breakfast (Conway, 1988)	36
3 year check – all	59
Ealing Health Authority estimate 1988	50

* insufficient data

women. Children suffer a high rate of infections, accidents and developmental delay; 16% of babies born to mothers in bed and breakfast accommodation are of low birth weight (<2500 g), compared to a national average of <10% in a survey in 1988 (Conway *et al.*, 1988).

Families in bed and breakfast accommodation not only suffer increased morbidity because of poverty but also because of poor access to existing health facilities. This is partly because increased mobility means that appointments and referrals arrive after they have moved on. Prejudice from service staff in the health service, local authority and DSS, together with inflexible rules, compound existing ignorance of available facilities in a strange locality. Our experience of working with families living in hotels and hostels suggests that this observation is still valid. Feelings of isolation, and marital and emotional problems, depression and postnatal depression are common. In Ealing 1989/90 we also found among children whilst routine visiting:

- Diarrhoea and vomiting requiring hospital admission.
- Asthma requiring hospital admission.
- Untreated squint.
- Undiagnosed developmental delay.
- Varying degrees of deafness.
- Lice, scabies, bedbugs, fleas.
- Speech problems requiring referral to speech therapy.
- Behaviour problems requiring referral to child guidance.

- Small for dates (5 lb) baby discharged to an unheated room in January with no change of baby clothes.
- Babies and children failing to thrive, requiring referral to paediatric clinic.
- Uncompleted immunization courses.
- Missed developmental checks.
- Respiratory infections.
- Falls and head injuries requiring attendance at the accident and emergency departments.
- Foot infections and thrush.
- Measles, mumps, chicken pox, influenza.
- Handicapped children and adults with no involvement of other services.
- Safety issues, i.e. drugs left in reach of children, rat poison left in reach of children in kitchen, open doors to street, unsafe playspace around hotels, three cases of molestation where children were playing unsupervised in corridors, bullying of children by other residents, and inadequate stairgates and banisters.
- Children on the 'at risk' register without allocated social workers.

In adults we found:

- Somalian mother discharged five days postnatally after inversion of uterus and 1000 ml post partum haemorrhage, without any money, clothes, equipment or ability to speak English.
- Single, blind Somalian man placed in hotel, who had epilepsy, hemiplegia and could not speak English; he later had an operation for a brain tumour.
- Clinical depression, schizophrenia and severe postnatal depression.
- Arthritis and back pain following epidural anaesthesia.
- Lack of antenatal care.
- 16 year olds receiving no antenatal care.
- Marital problems, including violence.
- Diarrhoea and vomiting.
- Respiratory infections, lice, bedbugs and scabies.

All families had problems with overcrowding, lack of playspace, difficult cooking and washing facilities, sharing bathrooms and toilets, difficulty in getting registered with a GP and receiving home visits by GP.

Although most of these families had a GP, many were not being treated for these problems. The disabled were getting no support services and the health visitor was the only professional seeking out the needs of this group and mobilizing support and making referrals.

It should be remembered that the characteristics of homeless populations change as boroughs change their placement policies. The findings of this study for the year 1989/90 may not be valid for 1993 and should be interpreted with caution in different populations.

Conclusion

When families are highly mobile and living in hostel or hotel accommodation, health issues get relegated down the list of priorities. Families may get trapped in a cycle of neglect, where preventative health care is missed, ensuring most problems have become crises by the time they are treated. The health visitor is the *only* health professional seeking out health needs and offering a non-stigmatizing service to this disadvantaged group.

Although the major reports on primary health care and the homeless emphasize the importance of encouraging families to use existing health facilities, in practice many families do have problems using them and many GPs refuse to do home visits. The health visitors in the homeless families unit seem ideally placed to pilot a nurse practitioner role with limited prescribing rights.

Purchasers are becoming clearer about their new role in specifying services and agreeing contracts with the providers of health care for their populations. When residents do not originate from the host authority, it is predictable that there will be increasing reluctance to provide a service and there needs to be a recognition of the health needs of homeless people within their area. For further information, two guides to commissioning services for the homeless have been published by Access to Health, a short term joint initiative of the King's Fund and the Thames Regional Health Authorities (Access to Health, 1992 a and b).

It has been suggested to us that the work we were doing with these families was not health visiting, but neither was it social work. From our viewpoint, one starts by accepting one of the most academically well founded results from social epidemiology and medical sociology over the last twenty years – that increased mobidity and mortality is inversely related to class position (Townsend & Davidson, 1982; Whitehead, 1987; Smith & Jacobson, 1988).

'Most recent data show marked differences in mortality rates between the occupational classes, for both sexes and at all ages. At birth and in the first month of life, twice as many babies of "unskilled manual" parents die as babies of professional parents ... Available data on chronic sickness tend to parallel those on mortality.'

Townsend and Davidson, 1982

The authors of The Black Report suggested changes in health and social services such as increased child and family benefits, based on the assumption that the battle against inequalities in health had to be placed within the wider strategy of social equity and justice. This overtly political framework for tackling variations in the distribution of health and disease did not find favour with a government concerned to emphasize individual responsibility and behaviour as the main determinants of health, and the £2 billion proposals suggested by The Black Report have never been implemented.

This viewpoint is also conspicuous by its absence from a recent government policy document, *The Health of the Nation* (Department of Health, 1992), which sets out targets and priorities for the health services. Here, health differentials are 'in part accounted for by differences in risk behaviour'. This ideological refusal to accept that poverty is a major cause of ill health means that health programmes emphasizing lifestyle changes can only have limited success, because lifestyle changes are constrained by poor housing and poverty. Furthermore, while attempts to change individual behaviour receive high levels of support from professionals, these methods are relatively ineffective (Stone, 1989).

Marxist critics will not be surprised at this official viewpoint, seeing it as the view of those who seek to promote the powerful interests of capital in society over the interests of the poor who suffer disproportionately the effects of poverty and environmentally induced poor health, and who have the least resources to change their circumstances for the better (Navarro, 1978). As Tuckett (1979) pointed out, the distribution of power and authority in society will always influence views about health and illness and the policies and strategies used. But it is also important to mention that politicians only partly control the agenda. Inequalities in health are not high on the public agenda, possibly because many people believe that health is one area where we are all equal (Blaxter, 1990).

It is important not to overemphasize the deterministic nature of structural influences on health, i.e. not all people who are poor get sick. It would be a very pessimistic view of society that said human beings are totally constrained by circumstances and never have the opportunity to challenge them.

Although the evidence supporting the impact of poverty and ill health is undisputed, what is still open to debate is the dynamics between structural and behavioural factors. What we need to consider is how much health workers can realistically achieve, bearing in mind these powerful constraints (Blaxter, 1983) and we need to find creative ways of working to achieve these aims.

References

Access to Health (1992a) *How to Count Your Homeless Population.* Access to Health, London.

Access to Health (1992b) *Purchasing and Poverty: A Guide to Commissioning Health Services for Homeless People.* Access to Health, London.

Audit Commission (1989) Housing the Homeless. Audit Commission, London.

Bayswater Hotel Homelessness Project (1987) *Speaking for Ourselves.* Bayswater Hotel Homelessness Project, London.

Blaxter, M. (1983) Health services as a defence against the consequences of poverty in industrialised societies. *Soc. Sci. Med.,* **17**, (16) 1139–48.

Blaxter, M. (1990) *Health and Lifestyles.* Routledge, London.

Boyer, J. (1986) Homelessness from a health visitor's point of view. *Health Visitor,* 59, 332–3.

British Medical Association (1989) *Homeless Families and Their Health.* Health Visitors Association and General Medical Services Committee, London.

Connelly, I., Roderick, P. & Victor, C. (1990) Health service planning for the homeless population. *Public Health,* 104, 109–16.

Conway, J., Cole-Hamilton, I. & Durward, L. (1988) Prescription for Poor Health: the Crisis for Homeless Families. London Housing Aid Centre, London Food Commission, Maternity Alliance.

Department of Health (1992) *The Health of the Nation.* Her Majesty's Stationery Office, London.

Drennan, V. & Stearn, J. (1986) Health visitors and homeless families. *Health Visitor,* 59, 340–2.

Ealing Health Authority (1990) *Ealing Annual Health Report.*

Ealing Local Authority (1982) *Census Digest of Population for Ealing.*

Ealing Local Authority (1989) *Job Centre.*

Evans, A. & Duncan, S. (1988) *Responding to Homelessness: Local Authority Policy and Practice.* Her Majesty's Stationery Office.

Frankenburg, W.K. & Dodds, J.B. (1973) *Denver Development Screening Test.* University of Colorado Medical Centre.

Hayden, C. & Bose, R. (1991) *Picking up the Pieces?* Social Services Research Information Unit Report No. 19, Portsmouth Polytechnic.

Health Visitors Association (1989) *Health Visiting and Homelessness,* pack 1. Special Interest Group for Homelessness, Health Visitors Association, London.

Housing Act 1985. Her Majesty's Stationery Office, London.

Housing (Homeless Persons) Act 1977 (1983) *Code of guidance (England and Wales)*. Her Majesty's Stationery Office, London.

LHAC (1989) *Homeless and Housing Need in London*. London Housing Aid Centre.

London Housing Forum (1988) *Speaking Out: Report of the London Housing Enquiry*. London Housing Forum, London.

London Research Centre (1988) *Homelessness And The Use Of Temporary Accommodation in London*. Report of Bed and Breakfast Information Exchange Survey.

Morton, S. (1990) Health and homelessness. *Health Visitor*, **63**(6) 191–3.

Navarro, V. (1978) *Class Struggle, the State and Medicine*. Martin Robertson, London.

Paterson, C. & Roderick, P. (1990) Obstetric outcome in homeless women. *Brit. Med. J.* **301**, 263–6.

Popay, J., Dhooge, Y. & Shipman, C. (1986) Unemployment and health: What Role for Health and Social Services? *Research Report No 3*, Health Education Council, London.

Roof (1989a) Waving or Drowning. *Roof*, May/June.

Roof (1989b) At Home With Fear. *Roof*, July/Aug.

Sandall, J. (1990) Homeless Families and Health in Ealing in 1989. *Ealing Health Authority*.

Smith, A. & Jacobson, B. (Eds) (1988) The Nation's Health – a Strategy for the 1990s. King's Fund, London.

Social Trends 21 (1991) Her Majesty's Stationery Office, London.

Stone, I. (1989) Upside down prevention. *Health Service Journal*, 99, 890–1.

Townsend, P. & Davidson, N. (1982) *The Black Report*. Penguin Books, London.

Tuckett, D. (1979) Choices for health education: a framework for decision making. In *Health Education Perspectives and Choices* (Ed. I. Sutherland). Allen Unwin, London.

Tudor Hart, J. (1971) The inverse care law. *The Lancet*, 1, 405–12.

Whitehead, M. (1987) *The Health Divide*. Health Education Council, London.

Chapter 12
Health Promotion and Cancer Care

Cancer represents a major health challenge. It is the second largest cause of death in the developed world with around 250 000 new cases diagnosed each year in the UK, and 160 000 people dying of the disease (Cancer Research Campaign, 1990). It is also a disease surrounded by myth, stigma and fear, considered by the general public and health care professionals alike as synonymous with death.

In recent years there has been an upsurge in public education campaigns at informing the public of how they can reduce their risks of dying from cancer, and there are mass screening programmes for cancers of the cervix and breast. These developments are positive for health promotion, but also present dilemmas for the lay public and for health carers since the disease remains feared more than any other conditions and screening and health promotion campaigns can raise anxiety and fear. They have also presented dilemmas about how best to treat cancers diagnosed at a very early stage, particularly as cancer therapy is by definition aggressive, has side effects and long term sequelae, and can be mutilating. In addition, it is known that receiving a diagnosis of cancer can have profound and negative psychological effects.

There is also the wider issue of promoting health in the situation in which individuals are diagnosed as having cancer. There is much health promotion activity required to assist individuals and their families to cope with the diagnosis of cancer, and to assist in decision making about whether to accept aggressive cancer treatment and participate in clinical trials of new therapies. Much work is required to support patients undergoing cancer treatment which has physical and psychological side effects and sequelae. With developments in the treatment of cancer, there is also now a great need for health promoting activity among the survivors of cancer, as they attempt to rebuild their lives in the months and years following treatment. Even in the context of palliative care and end-stage, incurable disease, the primary aim of care and treatment is to maximize and enhance life quality in its broadest sense.

This chapter will explore the range of issues that health promotion and cancer raises, will confront the many dilemmas facing health policy makers and health care professionals, and will explore the particular contribution that nursing can make to this area.

Cancer as a health problem

Cancer is a lay term that encompasses many different diseases; consequently the collection of diseases it represents is frequently misunderstood. The lay conception of the disease is extraordinarily powerful, to the extent that even those expert in the care of patients with the disease are personally influenced by its lay meaning.

The group of diseases termed cancer share common characteristics of growth, spread and behaviour. The link between them is of abnormal and uncoordinated growth of tissue, which can be benign or malignant. Malignant or cancerous tumours are characterized by their ability to infiltrate and disrupt or destroy normal tissue with which they come into contact, and also to metastasize, or disseminate, to areas distant from the site of original growth (Gowing & Fisher, 1988). With cancer, each separate disease entity is represented by the site at which the cancer

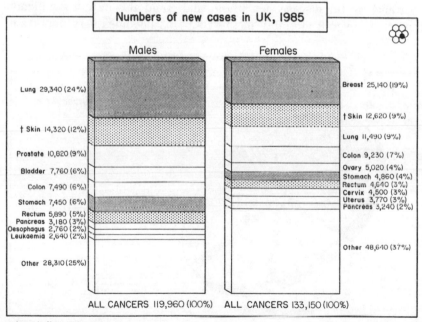

† excluding melanoma

Fig. 12.1 Facts on cancer. (Reprinted with permission from Cancer Research Campaign Fact Sheet, 1989.)

originates. So for example, cancer of the lung arises from the epithelial tissue of the lung, and the leukaemias develop from cellular proliferations in the bone marrow. It is because of cancer's ability to spread and metastasize, that it can invade and disrupt the functioning of all the major organs and is a life threatening disease.

As has already been stated, more than a quarter of a million people are diagnosed as having cancer each year, and one in three people will develop cancer at some point in their lives (Cancer Research Campaign, 1990). This puts cancer as second only to cardiovascular disease in terms of disease incidence and mortality. Relatively few cancer sites, though, account for the majority of individuals diagnosed with the disease, with lung cancer accounting for 16% of all new cases and breast cancer accounting for 10%. Cancer is in the main a disease of middle and old age with 70% of cancers occurring in those aged over 60 years. Fig. 12.1 shows the incidence rates of the ten most common cancers in the UK.

Four cancer sites account for over 50% of cancer deaths (Fig. 12.2). Of these, cancer of the lung accounts for 25% of all cancer deaths. It is interesting to note that the cancers responsible for the greater proportion of the mortality are also, with the exception of cancer of the skin, among the most common cancer sites. Any reduction in deaths from each of these four cancer sites would therefore have a major impact on mortality for the disease as a whole, and could also have a significant impact on overall mortality in the UK. This becomes very important

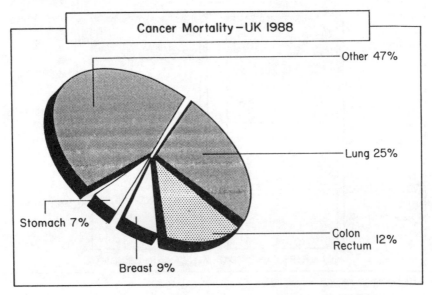

Fig. 12.2 Facts on cancer. (Reprinted with permission from Cancer Research Campaign Fact Sheet, 1989.)

when one considers the causative factors for cancers of different sites, and also when examining possibilities for cancer prevention. Nowhere is this more true that in the case of lung cancer, where between 80% and 90% of lung cancer cases are attributable to smoking (Cancer Research Campaign, 1992).

When examining cancer as a health problem, the consideration of disease incidence and mortality rates in the population only gives a limited picture of the disease. The length of survival from diagnosis of the disease is also important, since the proportion of people surviving a given period of time with cancers of different sites varies considerably. A scrutiny of rate and duration of survival will give an indication of the curability of each disease site. With cancer it is usual to compare this by examining five year survival figures across disease sites, from the time of diagnosis. Figure 12.3 shows the five year survival rates for the ten most common cancers. From this it is possible to identify cancers where survival rates are very high, such as cancers of the skin (excluding melanoma), and cancers where the outlook is much poorer, such as cancer of the lung where the five year survival rate for the disease is only 8%. Around 40% of all cancer patients will be cured of their disease with treatment (Department of Health, 1991).

Of great importance, though, is also the stage of the disease at diagnosis. Cancers identified at an early stage, when the primary tumour is limited in size and before the cancer has had a chance to spread to other areas of the body, is much more likely to be curable. This is particularly evident in, for example, cancer of the cervix, when early stage disease,

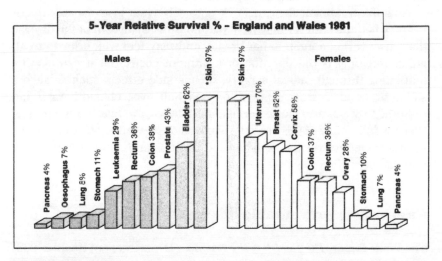

Fig. 12.3 Facts on cancer. (Reprinted with permission from Cancer Research Campaign Fact Sheet, 1989.)

picked up before the disease has become invasive, is curable with treatment, whereas when women present with the disease at an advanced stage, five year survival drops to around 20% (Cancer Research Campaign, 1989).

Treatment for cancer is complex and intense and is costly for both health care providers and for cancer sufferers who may have to take considerable time off work to undergo therapy, and may also find themselves penalized after treatment is finished by employers, life insurers and building societies. In the last 20 years cancer treatment has undergone a revolution through the use of multi-modality treatments and more recently the refinement of such treatment to reduce side-effects; these developments have brought about significant reductions in mortality for a number of cancers.

Multi-modality treatment means that treatment is not confined to the surgical removal of the tumour, for example lumpectomy or mastectomy for breast cancer. It is now known that in many cancers, micro-metastases, too small to be detected, are likely to have reached distant parts of the body; therefore treatment is aimed at eradicating the primary tumour, and also at destroying any micro-metastatic deposits which may be present in the body. For this reason surgery will often be combined with chemotherapy, radiotherapy and possibly hormonal and biological therapies. For example, the treatment of breast cancer frequently involves surgical removal of the breast lump, by lumpectomy, radiotherapy to the chest wall to prevent local recurrence of the disease, and up to six months of chemotherapy and/or taking of anti-oestrogen drugs for several years (Donaldson *et al.*, 1986).

Thus the treatment for cancer is aggressive and lasts for months or years, when the sufferer may have had no other symptom of the disease than discovering a lump in her breast, and may feel well prior to treatment. Not only is the duration of treatment costly but it can also be mutilating through radical surgery, or has side effects such as severe sickness, bone marrow suppression and hair loss; chemotherapy and radiotherapy can also cause permanent damage and loss of functioning. Clearly if all or any of this could be avoided or prevented, it would have a significant effect on the well-being of a substantial sub-group of the population.

Cancer as a preventable disease

The White Paper, *The Health of the Nation*, (Department of Health, 1992) has identified cancer as a target area for the reduction in morbidity and mortality, through the new National Health Service strategy for health.

Three cancer sites have been identified as having potential for a large scale reduction in mortality: lung cancer (to be reduced by 30% in men and 15% in women by the year 2000, through reducing smoking), breast cancer (25% reduction in mortality) and cervical cancers, through improving the uptake of existing screening programmes. The central place that cancer has in the health strategy of this country demands that the potential for cancer to be preventable requires some examination.

A scrutiny of cancer incidence figures worldwide quickly leads to the conclusion that there are great variations in the pattern of cancer incidence. For example, breast cancer, which is common in the UK, is relatively rare in Japan where cancer of the stomach is the most prevalent cancer site; and liver cancer, endemic in African countries, is rare in Western ones (Doll & Peto, 1981). In addition, studies of migrant populations suggest that they demonstrate the cancer incidence pattern of the country to which they migrate, rather than their country of origin. For this reason there is powerful evidence of a substantial environmental influence on the development of cancer, and this may be more important than genetic or intrinsic factors (Doll & Peto, 1981). Such evidence has led Doll & Peto to conclude that 75% of cancers might be avoidable.

What is much more complex, however, is deciphering the causative factors and mechanisms in the development of cancer. Yet it is an understanding of these which will assist in the development of cancer prevention strategies. It is known that carcinogenesis, the steps through which normal cells become cancerous, is a multi-step process and it has been described by Archer (1987) as follows:

(1) Exposure of a cell to the carcinogen causes initiation, an irreversible and normally rapid process causing permanent changes in the DNA of cells.

(2) Tumour formation is promoted in initiated tissues through a series of usually reversible steps. This occurs following initiation, during a period of latency spanning many years, before cancerous cells appear. Factors which promote the development of pre-neoplastic cells may be the same or different from initiating factors. For example, alcohol does not produce cancer in animal models but is a potent co-carcinogen, increasing the risk of cancer of the mouth, larynx and oesophagus in smokers (Meyskens, 1992).

(3) Progression occurs as the cancer cells become progressively more malignant. The factors which cause pre-neoplastic cells to become neoplastic is uncertain, and pre-neoplastic conditions can spontaneously regress. Pre-neoplastic cells can be identified using clinical observation or investigation techniques, whereas the

identification of the earlier stages of carcinogenesis requires sophisticated laboratory techniques. This also means that the process of carcinogenesis is difficult to detect for a large proportion of the process of cancer development.

The factors which are known to cause initiation and promotion of normal cells are complex. Chromosomal abnormalities predisposing to cancer may be inherited or caused by carcinogenic substances such as asbestos or benzene, or for example viruses or exposure to radiation. Doll & Peto (1981) have identified the determinants of who will and will not develop cancer as:

(1) Genetic – an inherited predisposition to develop cancer.
(2) Environmental factors that an individual is exposed to in the womb, during childhood or in adult life.
(3) Luck.

They have also detailed the percentage of cancer deaths which can be attributed to different causative factors (Table 12.1). The epidemiological work undertaken by authors such as Sir Richard Doll has been instrumental in establishing the links between cancer-causing substances or behaviours and subsequent cancer development. For

Table 12.1 Proportions of cancer deaths attributed to various different factors. (Reprinted with permission of Oxford University Press, from Doll, R. & Peto, R. (1981).) *The Causes of Cancer*, Oxford Medical Publications, Oxford.

Factor or class of factors	% of all cancer deaths	
	Best estimate	Range of acceptable estimates
Tobacco	30	25–40
Alcohol	3	2–4
Diet	35	10–70
Food additives	<1	–5–2
Reproductive and sexual behaviour	7	1–13
Occupation	4	2–8
Pollution	2	<1–5
Industrial products	<1	<1–2
Medicines and medical procedures	1	0.5–3
Geophysical factors	3	2–4
Infection	10?	1–?
Unknown	?	?

example, they established the link between smoking and lung cancer (Doll & Peto 1976).

Research on environmental factors which are known to be either initiators or promoters of cancer has permitted the development of key strategies for cancer avoidance, which can be used in health education campaigns aimed at reducing mortality from cancer. In 1989 the European Commission's Europe Against Cancer programme launched a ten point code for avoiding cancer, with the aim of reducing mortality from cancer in Europe by 15% by the year 2000, through changing lifestyle and habits and detecting cancers early. The Cancer Education Co-ordinating Group of the United Kingdom and Republic of Ireland have produced a leaflet detailing the code and the rationale behind each point. A copy of it is shown in Fig. 12.4, and represents a useful guide to health promotion advice for cancer avoidance.

Much of the current research effort in cancer prevention and treatment is increasingly being invested in attempts at identifying the genes responsible for cancer development, and in developing understanding of the genetic defects that occur during the disease process (Cavenee *et al.*, 1991). While this work is at an experimental and embryonic stage, it will soon be possible to identify individuals at risk of developing cancer by examining their genetic make-up. This will dramatically change approaches to screening for cancer, and will have great implications for health promoters, since screening and treatment efforts may be concentrated on individuals and their family members identified to be at high risk, and may even in time make mass screening and public education programmes redundant. But great thought and care will be required about how to inform and work with individuals considered to be at risk.

Cancer care as a context for health promotion

The scope for health promotion in cancer care is enormous, not only because it has been established that many cancers are avoidable, but also because of the nature of the disease itself, of cancer treatment and of the chronic, degenerative nature of many kinds of cancer.

Health promotion must always address the meaning of health and illness within society; nowhere is this more important than in cancer care. Cancer as a disease evokes a very powerful and emotive image in society; Sontag (1979) argues that society has a distorted image of cancer so that it is regarded not simply as a fatal disease but has become a metaphor for suffering and is viewed as synonymous with death itself, and a death that involves much pain and suffering. This is in direct

AVOIDING CANCER

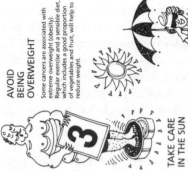

THE EUROPEAN CODE

a **10** point code

'Europe against Cancer' is a campaign to encourage people to take action to reduce the number of deaths from cancer by 15%. Countries in the European Community are publicising

based on current knowledge about prevention and early detection. The code has been approved by the European Community's Committee of Experts. This leaflet, funded by the Community and HEA, contains the ten points from the European Code.

FIRM GUIDELINES

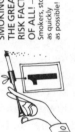

1

SMOKING IS THE GREATEST RISK FACTOR OF ALL! –
Smokers, stop as quickly as possible!

Cigarette smoking causes a third of all cancer deaths. At least 90% of lung cancers are due to smoking. Smoking also increases the risk of cancer of the mouth, voice-box (larynx), gullet (oesophagus), bladder and some other cancers. The longer a person smokes the more dangerous it becomes, so starting to smoke when young seriously increases the risk to health. The good news is that the risk begins to fall as soon as a smoker stops smoking.

There is now evidence that non-smokers' health can be damaged by constant exposure to smoke from other people's cigarettes (called 'passive smoking'). Chewing or sucking tobacco is not a safe habit – it can lead to cancer of the mouth.

GO EASY ON THE ALCOHOL

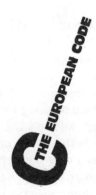

2

Drinking too much alcohol has been linked to about 3% of cancers, particularly those of the mouth, larynx, oesophagus and liver. If heavy drinkers also smoke, the risk becomes even higher.

A sensible limit is two or three pints of beer, (or the equivalent), two or three times a week – less if you are a woman. (One pint of beer is the equivalent of a double measure of spirits or two glasses of wine.)

AVOID BEING OVERWEIGHT

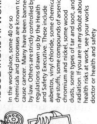

3

Some cancers are associated with extreme overweight (obesity). Regular exercise and a sensible diet, which includes a good proportion of vegetables and fruit, will help to reduce weight.

TAKE CARE IN THE SUN

4

Too much sun can cause skin cancer, so remember to protect your skin in the sun, especially during holidays abroad in hot countries. Tan slowly, avoid sunburn and use sun filter creams and lotions – lots and often.

You should take special care if you are fair-haired or have a skin which always burns in the sun or tans little and slowly.

OBSERVE THE HEALTH AND SAFETY REGULATIONS AT WORK

5

In the workplace, some 40 or so chemicals and processes are known to cause cancer. Many have been banned by law. Others are strictly controlled by regulations drawn up by the Health and Safety Executive. These include asbestos, vinyl chloride, some chemical dye stuffs, some compounds of arsenic, chromium and nickel, some wood dusts, some types of tar and soot, and radiation. If you are in any doubt about health risks at work, see your works doctor or health and safety representative.

GENERAL GUIDELINES

CUT DOWN ON FATTY FOODS

It is known that in Western countries, where people usually eat a lot of meat, butter and other dairy products, there is a higher risk of breast and bowel cancer as well as other diseases, like coronary heart disease. A sensible diet can reduce this risk. Eat lean meat, try fish or chicken instead of red meat. Bake or grill instead of frying. Try skimmed or semi-skimmed milk instead of full-cream milk.

EAT PLENTY OF FRESH FRUIT AND VEGETABLES AND OTHER FOODS CONTAINING FIBRE

There is some evidence that foods rich in carotenoids (pro-vitamin A), vitamin C and fibre may give protection against cancer. Food containing fibre may actually protect against cancer of the bowel. Fibre is found in fresh fruit and vegetables, but mostly in wholegrain cereals and bread. Most fruit and vegetables contain the necessary vitamins and vitamin A is also present in fish. Natural foods are the best way to obtain these vitamins and fibre.

SEE YOUR DOCTOR IF THERE IS ANY UNEXPLAINED CHANGE IN YOUR NORMAL HEALTH WHICH LASTS FOR MORE THAN TWO WEEKS

Most symptoms are unlikely to mean cancer, but it is always worthwhile consulting your doctor if they persist. So if you notice a lump, a change in a skin mole, any unusual bleeding, or develop a persistent cough or hoarseness, a change in bowel habits or unexplained weight loss, see your doctor at once.

ESPECIALLY FOR WOMEN

HAVE A REGULAR CERVICAL SMEAR TEST

The smear test can detect abnormal changes in the cells of the neck of the womb (cervix) before cancer has actually developed and when the cure rate is very high. If cervical cancer can be detected and treated at an early stage, it too is curable. So every woman who is, or has been, sexually active should have a smear test every 3-5 years. If you have never had a smear test, or have not had one within the last five years, go to your doctor or family planning clinic and ask for one.

EXAMINE YOUR BREASTS MONTHLY
(Women over the age of 50 should be screened by mammography at regular intervals.)

Many doctors recommend that women should examine their own breasts each month. This should be done carefully. There are leaflets that tell you how. If you do notice any lumps, a dimple or puckering, or other changes, arrange to see your doctor at once. Remember, most lumps are not cancer but it's best to be sure.

The aim of screening is to detect breast cancer at the earliest possible stage. Treatment is then likely to be simpler and offer a better chance of cure.

The NHS is setting up breast screening clinics offering mammography (a type of X-ray which can show up very early changes in breast tissue). Women aged 50-64 will be invited for screening every three years. Any woman outside this age range and concerned about a breast problem, or any woman needing specific information, should seek her doctor's advice.

'EUROPE AGAINST CANCER' Campaign

This leaflet was produced by the Cancer Education Co-ordinating Group of the United Kingdom and Republic of Ireland.

Fig. 12.4 The Europe Against Cancer Code for Avoiding Cancer. (Reproduced with permission.)

contrast to the metaphors surrounding other diseases, such as cardio-
vascular disease which is associated with power, success and an easy,
pain free death (Donovan & Girton, 1984). Sontag (1988) argues that in
the United States beliefs about cancer are changing due to greater
openness about the disease, and cancer is being surpassed by AIDS as
the most feared disease, with its metaphor of plague. There is little
evidence to suggest that fear of cancer is changing in the UK and Europe.

Brooks (1979) in reviewing surveys of public attitudes towards cancer
concludes that 'one is left with the strong impression that cancer is seen
to be very threatening, the most dreaded of all diseases, rarely if ever
curable and largely unavoidable'. A more recent survey of public opinion
undertaken by Cancer Relief Macmillan Fund (1988) found that cancer is
still feared 'more than death itself' by a substantial proportion of the
population, and AIDS is only feared more than cancer among the
younger age groups.

This negative perception of cancer can be seen to affect health
behaviour. Delay in seeking medical attention for cancer is a frequent
problem. In a review of studies examining the problem of delay, Eddy &
Eddy (1984) concluded that between 25% and 75% of patients delayed
more than three months before seeking medical attention for symptoms
of cancer. The likelihood for an individual to put off visiting the doctor
was influenced by perceived risk, beliefs about likely benefit from
treatment, desire for reassurance, and the inconvenience of undergoing
diagnostic tests and procedures. It is still the case, for example, that a
minority of women ignore a lump in their breast until the cancer is a very
large fungating lesion, which is much more difficult to treat. There have
also been problems with women not taking up screening opportunities
for cancer of the cervix, particularly among lower socioeconomic
groups (Charny *et al.* 1987); the reasons for this are complex and not
solely due to fear of cancer, although this must play a part.

Health promotion needs to address how it can be best used to change
society's construction of cancer, so that a less negative view of the
disease is held and the value of treatment is recognized. This is a complex and difficult problem and much of the literature focuses on fostering positive attitudes towards cancer. Yet this would seem to be an
overly simplistic approach, since to some extent the popular conception
of cancer does reflect the fact that 50–60% of cancer sufferers will not be
cured of the disease. The message that needs to be conveyed to the
public is that the quality of living with cancer is improved with treatment,
and that this is the case even where the disease may not be curable. This,
however, is a subtle and difficult message to convey to a mass audience.
It is particularly important since, although the Health Belief Model
(Becker & Maiman, 1975) would suggest that fear is an important

motivator for taking preventative health action, in the case of cancer it would seem that the extent and depth of fear is so great that it immobilizes individuals and prevents them seeking help for symptoms of the disease (Brooks, 1979).

Health promotion in cancer care is not solely confined to the issue of educating the public on ways of avoiding cancer, or ensuring that all cancer patients receive optimum treatment for their disease at the earliest possible stage through screening and early detection methods. The chronic nature of cancer means that there is enormous potential for promoting optimum health and quality of life among patients with cancer and their families, at all stages of the disease.

Because of the diversity of need for health promotion in cancer care, the scope for it in this field is discussed below under the headings of primary, secondary and tertiary health promotion. Primary health promotion means the prevention of cancer; secondary health promotion is the early detection of disease; and tertiary health promotion is the amelioration of disease and treatment induced problems, and the enhancement of the quality of life of people with cancer.

The scope of health promotion in cancer care

Primary health promotion

It is clear from the negative image of cancer for society that promoting a more positive image and dispelling myths about the disease need to play a central role in action taken to prevent cancer. Nurses and other health care professionals have an important role to play in this. There are problems here, however, since a body of evidence exists which indicates that nurses and other health care professionals are themselves very pessimistic about the disease (Corner, 1988).

Elkind's (1981, 1982) survey of 785 nurses' beliefs about cancer led her to conclude that some nurses are likely to find it difficult to pass on anything other than an entirely negative view of the disease. Dawson's (1991) study of women undergoing treatment for cancer of the ovary found that GPs' failure to take women's symptoms seriously led to considerable delay in their cancer being diagnosed. It would seem that negative attitudes and a lack of knowledge on the part of health care professionals are an important contributory factor to the problem of cancer prevention and early detection. Health care professionals need help and education to examine their own belief systems and to develop their knowledge in this area (Corner & Wilson Barnett, 1992).

The focus of primary health promotion is to encourage the adoption of 'healthy lifestyles' in order to prevent the disease developing. In cancer care, research and knowledge are about 15 years behind that for cardiovascular disease prevention (Meyskens, 1992). Identifying the factors to avoid to prevent cancer are also much more complex than in cardiovascular disease, since as already mentioned cancer represents a collection of quite different diseases, each with different cancer-causing factors. This has made it much more difficult to identify the kind of code for cancer avoidance shown earlier.

There is an additional problem in that scientists researching the causative factors in every chronic disease could come up with different lifestyles that are most conducive to avoiding particular diseases. This could quickly become a self-defeating exercise if one has to select a 'healthy lifestyle' by choosing the disease one fears most. Fortunately there have so far been commonalities between lifestyles promoted for cardiovascular disease prevention and cancer prevention, such as reducing fat in the diet, avoiding obesity and stopping smoking. There are also problems in taking an overly didactic approach to conveying information aimed at preventing cancer, since people's lifestyles are bound up with their culture and their own personal history. It is unlikely that the threat of cancer in itself will change such behaviour.

Nurses and other health care professionals need to be clear about what messages they are giving their clients, and they have an important role to play in interpreting research and media scares on different carcinogenic substances, so that cancer avoidance efforts focus on those factors which are likely to cause the greatest reduction in cancer mortality. Of these, encouraging and assisting individuals to give up smoking is possibly the single most important health promoting action which can be taken. Research has demonstrated that with a modest amount of training, nurses can be very effective in assisting men and women to stop smoking by giving sympathetic help and advice. This, however, is most effective when nurses work in partnership with the individual, rather than taking on the role of 'preacher' (Macleod Clark *et al.*, 1989).

Secondary health promotion

Much of the emphasis on cancer prevention to date has focused on early detection, when the disease is at an early or pre-invasive stage. Two strategies exist here: first, raising the awareness of the public to early warning signs of cancer, so that they detect these themselves and come forward for treatment as early as possible; and second, developing methods of mass screening of the population so that cancers can be detected in asymptomatic individuals, who can then be offered curative treatment. However, as Chamberlain (1988) points out, great caution needs to be exercised when considering the development of screening services; it is not automatic that all cancers are amenable to this form of early detection, and careful cost-benefit analyses need to be undertaken to determine the value of such approaches. For example, there are cancers that are small but aggressive and will have metastasized at an early stage; therefore early detection and treatment of the cancer may not improve prognosis from the disease. Likewise, indolent forms of cancer may be amenable to early detection but if left untreated may not lead to fatal disease progression. The risk of false positive results and consequent treatment of healthy individuals, and the likelihood of members of the population participating in the screening, need also to be considered.

The viability of screening for cancer therefore does not solely depend on the technological ability to identify early stage cancers. An example of this can be seen in the case of lung cancer where screening tests are available, yet studies have not shown that early detection significantly decreases mortality from the disease (Chamberlain, 1988).

National screening programmes exist for cancers of the cervix and breast. Screening for cancer of the cervix through the cervical smear test includes women from the age of 20, who it is recommended should have the test every three to five years. However, while the screening test itself is known to provide protection from invasive cancer for two years following the test (MacGregor *et al.*, 1986), there has been no reduction in mortality from cervical cancer since the introduction of the screening service because many of those most at risk from developing the disease do not take up the opportunity of screening (Cancer Research Campaign, 1990).

In order to improve uptake GPs have been offered incentive payments for achieving targets for cervical screening of eligible women on their practice lists, and this seems to have had some effect in improving uptake rates (Eardley, 1992). This approach, though, is only likely to have a positive effect on mortality from cancer of the cervix if strenuous efforts are made to target 'at risk' groups of women – that is older women over the age of 40, those among the lower socio-economic groups and women from ethnic minorities rather than simply achieving the target proportion of women attending for smear tests.

The success of a screening programme must also be judged by the outcomes for women found to have a positive test. This is not only a question of rates of successful treatment, but also other sequelae which may result. Campion *et al.* (1988) found that women undergoing treatment for cervical intraepithelial neoplasia following abnormal smear, had psychosexual difficulties as a result, and McDonald *et al.* (1989)

found considerable anxiety about the possibility of having cancer, changes in body image and feelings of loss of attractiveness among such women. Other studies have highlighted women's fears of dying and of infertility after having a positive smear test (Possner & Vessey 1988). Since it is known that cervical screening diagnoses many more cases of intraepithelial disease than would be expected to develop invasive cancer (Cancer Research Campaign, 1990), over diagnoses may be causing unnecessary anxiety and psychosexual sequelae.

Breast cancer, as the commonest cancer in women, with one in 12 developing the disease at some point during their lives (Cancer Research Campaign, 1991), has been the focus of much debate and study with regard to the most effective methods of detecting it at as early a stage as possible. This culminated in 1988 in the introduction of a national breast cancer screening programme using mammography, for all women between the ages of 50 and 64 years, at three yearly intervals, following the Forrest Report (1986) recommendations. Mammography has the ability to detect breast lesions that are too small to be manually palpable or are at the carcinoma in situ stage. Randomized trials of mammography screening have been shown to reduce mortality from breast cancer by between 20% and 40% (Forrest, 1986).

The National Breast Screening Programme is run from regional centres using notification lists of eligible women, supplied by GPs. The service operates a call and recall system whereby women are personally invited to attend for screening, and informed of the result. Results of the service over one year to March 1991 showed that over 70% of women invited attended for screening, 7.1% of whom needed to be recalled for further investigation, and just over five women in every 1000 screened had a cancer detected. The uptake of this service has been good relative to cervical screening programmes (Cancer Research Campaign, 1991). The primary health care team play a pivotal role in promoting the screening service to eligible women, discussing with women the mammography procedure and talking over any anxieties women may have regarding screening.

While the National Breast Screening Programme has a very important aim of reducing mortality from breast cancer, as with cervical screening the initiation of such a service is not without consequences for women undergoing screening. Anxiety among women who are recalled for assessment following the detection of an abnormality, and particularly among those who undergo biopsy is likely to be very high. (One in three women following mammography will have cancer – Austoker & Humphreys, 1988).

In recent years the assessment of breast lumps has advanced to the stage where the majority of women can know the likelihood of their breast lump being cancerous at the time of assessment (Donaldson *et al.*, 1986), and this has helped reduce the intense anxiety experienced while undergoing biopsy and during the consequent time lag in waiting for results of the histological examination of biopsy tissue (Maguire *et al.*, 1978). The detection of abnormalities in the breast tissue that are not identifiable by manual palpation through mammography, however, also means that these are more likely to require biopsy, and women may have to wait several days for the result.

It is known that around 25% of women diagnosed with breast cancer will have psychological symptoms serious enough to require treatment (Maguire *et al.*, 1978); what is not yet known are the psychological consequences of screen-detected breast cancers. While women may be reassured that their cancer has been detected at an early stage, they may not also have gone through the more gradual process of identifying a breast lump themselves, and seeking attention for it.

The National Breast Screening Programme is a recent development and only includes women within a narrow age band. Also, since to date 90% of breast cancers are detected by women themselves (Faulder, 1992), much energy has been devoted to the question of early detection methods which encourage women to examine their own breasts. Prior to the introduction of breast screening, the early detection for breast cancer relied on teaching women breast self examination – the regular, systematic self examination of both breasts.

A number of studies have examined the efficacy of such an approach in detecting breast lumps, but have come up with equivocal results and identify a low rate of compliance (Holmes, 1987). This led the Department of Health to issue new guidelines regarding the early detection of breast cancer. These suggest that women, especially those over 40, should be aware of their breasts and what is normal about the feel and look of them during the menstrual cycle, and should report to their doctor without delay any changes in: the outline; shape or size of the breast; puckering or dimpling of the skin; any lump or thickening in the breast or armpit; any flaking of the skin; discharge from the nipple or any unusual pain or discomfort.

Nurses should play an active role in informing and teaching women in their care about breast awareness and in discussing with women any worries or concerns they may have about their breasts or the possibility of discovering a breast lump, bearing in mind that nine out of every 10 breast lumps are benign (Donaldson *et al.* 1986). Similarly men, particularly those under 40, should be encouraged to be aware that any swelling or lump in their testicles could be a sign of testicular cancer which is a less common but very treatable form of cancer (Pownall 1986).

Tertiary health promotion

Once cancer is diagnosed, many opportunities arise for the promotion of health and well-being. The whole of practice in cancer care is arguably working towards the relief of disease and treatment-induced needs and symptoms, and maximizing quality of life, regardless of whether an individual's disease is curable. It is beyond the scope of this chapter to give a full discussion of the range of opportunities for tertiary health promotion. Instead it would seem appropriate to discuss some issues which are highly pertinent to this concept.

It is now well known that the impact of receiving a diagnosis of cancer is devastating and requires significant adjustments to be made on the part of the sufferer as well as their family and friends (Weisman & Worden, 1976). Because of the association of cancer with inevitable death, the crisis of diagnosis is also about facing one's own mortality, even if the cancer is potentially curable. Most people want open and honest communication about their disease and future, although in the past there has been much debate as to whether this is detrimental for patients with cancer (McIntosh, 1974).

The arguments over whether to tell an individual that they have cancer have largely given way to discussions over the extent to which individuals with cancer should be involved in making informed choices about different treatments, and their involvement in clinical research trials since much cancer treatment is also experimental. Empowering individuals in such a way could certainly be considered a health promoting activity, although it is known that individuals differ in the extent to which they want to be involved in decision making about treatment. Some want to be allowed to participate fully while others may feel the need to place themselves in their doctor's hands, and this may be a powerful coping strategy (Rowland & Holland, 1989). Clearly health promotion in this area calls for great sophistication and sensitivity on the part of health carers.

One of the most important health promoting activities for individuals with cancer is to encourage them to talk over their feelings and fears about their disease, and to provide them with honest answers to their questions, providing them with information regarding treatment choices and with assistance in deciding what kind of partnership they want with the health care team. This partnership is one that is likely to exist for many months or years, and therefore may also change and develop over time.

Treatment for cancer is aggressive, lengthy and may involve mutilating surgery; radiotherapy and chemotherapy cause long term physical effects and may have long term consequences for fertility and sexual functioning (Tross & Holland, 1989). Because of this there has been increasing recognition of the need to carefully examine treatments in relation to their effects on quality of life and not solely on their ability to extend survival with the disease. In addition, because of the large numbers of people with cancer living with the disease for long periods of time, and the increasing number of people cured of the disease, the needs of 'cancer survivors' are now being recognized. Based on the work of Maher (1982) and Tross & Holland (1989), outline interventions for cancer survivors from the time of diagnosis to optimal rehabilitation are shown in Table 12.2.

A final and important concept in tertiary health promotion in cancer care is that of palliative care, i.e. providing continuing care and support, symptom control, rehabilitation and support and respite services for relatives and carers. Care therefore is aimed at maximizing the indi-

Table 12.2 Interventions to assist cancer survivors' adjustment. (Reprinted with permission of Oxford University Press, from Tross, S. & Holland, J.C. (1989). Psychological Sequelae in Cancer Survivors. In Holland, J.C. and Rowland, J.H. (eds) *Handbook of Psycho-oncology.* Oxford University Press, Oxford.

Adjustment Situation	Types of Intervention
At time of diagnosis	Honesty about diagnosis and possible delayed treatment effects.
	Opportunity for sperm banking prior to treatment, when infertility is anticipated.
	Sense of alliance with doctor about treatment.
On completion of treatment	Anticipation of increased anxiety in the immediate period after completion of treatment.
	Anticipation of no longer being 'a patient' and the reduction of special support and concern.
	Adjustment to physical side effects of treatment.
Re-entry in early survival	Counselling about how to deal with expectations of others: family, friends, workplace.
	Counselling to deal with personal feelings of increased anxiety about self-adequacy and future health.
	Help for family to prevent overprotection.
	Practical advice and support from veteran patient(s) with same illness.
Extended and permanent survival	Monitoring of physical and mental state by same medical staff (checking development milestones in children).
	Early referral for evaluation for signs of psychological distress.
	Becoming a veteran patient and helping others (promotes mastery).

vidual's functional potential and quality of life. While palliative care has grown out of the hospice movement, and therefore has focused predominantly on advanced cancer and the needs of the dying, it is felt that it should be introduced as early as possible in the course of the disease and certainly during the active treatment phase.

The role of nursing

The potential for health promotion in cancer care is clearly enormous and ranges from fostering a more positive view of the disease in society through to promoting lifestyles which reduce cancer risk; encouraging the uptake of services aimed at the early detection of cancer; and working towards promoting the highest quality of life possible among people who have been diagnosed with cancer, are undergoing treatment or who are survivors of the disease.

While there are many opportunities for health promotion, these also present dilemmas to nurses and other health carers as to where to concentrate their efforts. First and foremost all health care practitioners need to examine their own attitudes and beliefs about the disease so that they are conveying an approach which is optimistic and at the same time realistic for that individual and their particular situation.

Nurses also need to invest their health promoting activity in areas where they may have greatest effect; the message of the ten point code for avoiding cancer is valuable here. Informing and encouraging individuals to come forward for screening is an important role for nurses, as is the need to recognize the detrimental effects that such procedures may have on individuals, particularly those whose tests prove positive.

Above all, nurses need to be sensitive to the needs of individuals who are in the process of being diagnosed as having cancer, who are undergoing treatment or who have recurrent or advanced disease, and to work towards promoting the optimum quality of life for them – much of which entails using communication skills therapeutically – and providing supportive care and symptom management.

References

Archer, M.C. (1987) Chemical Carcinogenesis. In *The Basic Science of Oncology.* (Eds I.F. Tannock & R.P. Hill) Pergamon Press, New York.

Austoker, J. & Humphreys, J. (1988) *Breast Cancer Screening. Practical Guides for General Practice 6.* Oxford University Press.

Becker, M.M. & Maiman, B.A. (1975) Sociobehavioural determinents of compliance with and medical care recommendations. *Medical Care,* **13,** 10–24.

Brooks, A. (1979) Public and professional attitudes towards cancer: a view from Great Britain. *Cancer Nursing.* **2** (6) 453–60.

Campion, M.J., Brown, J.R., McCance, D.J., Atia, W., Edwards, R., Cuzick, J. & Singer, A. (1988) Psychosexual trauma of an abnormal cervical smear. *Brit. J. of Obstetrics and Gynaecology,* **95,** 175–81.

Cancer Relief Macmillan Fund (1988) *Public Attitudes and Knowledge of Cancer in the UK.* Unpublished Research Report.

Cancer Research Campaign (1990) *Fact sheets 1.1–1.3.* London.

Cancer Research Campaign (1990) *Fact sheets: Cervical Cancer Screening 13.1–13.5.* London.

Cancer Research Campaign (1991) *Fact sheets: Breast Cancer Screening 7.1–7.5.* London.

Cancer Research Campaign (1992) *Fact sheets: Lung Cancer and Smoking 11.1–11.5.* London.

Cavenee W.K., Ponder, B. & Solomon, E. (1991) Genetics and Cancer. *European Journal of Cancer,* **27** (12) 1706–7.

Chamberlain, J. (1988) Screening for Early Detection of Cancer. In *Oncology for Nurses and Health Care Professionals* (eds R. Tiffany & P. Pritchard) 2nd edn. Vol. 1. Harper and Row, Beaconsfield.

Charny, M.C., Farrow, S.C. & Lewis, P.A. (1987) Who is using cervical cancer screening services? *Health Trends.* **19,** 4.

Corner, J.L. (1988) Assessment of nurses' attitudes towards cancer: a critical review of research methods. *J. of Adv. Nurs.,* **13,** 640–8.

Corner, J.L. & Wilson-Barnett, J. (1992) The newly registered nurse and the cancer patient: an educational evaluation. *Int. J. of Nurs. Stud.,* **29,** (2) 177–90.

Dawson, T. (1991) Patients' Perceptions Following Treatment for Ovarian Cancer. Unpublished M.Sc. dissertation, University of Surrey.

Department of Health (1992) *The Health of the Nation.* A Consultative Document for Health in England. Her Majesty's Stationery Office, London.

Doll, R. & Peto, R. (1976) Mortality in relation to smoking: 20 years' observations on male British doctors. *Brit. Med. J.,* **2,** 1525–36.

Doll, R. & Peto, R. (1981) The Causes of Cancer. *Oxford Medical,* Oxford.

Donaldson, M. *et al.* (1986) Consensus development conference: treatment of primary breast cancer. *Brit. Med. J.,* **293,** 946–7.

Donovan, M.I. & Girton, S.E. (1984) *Cancer Care Nursing* (2nd edn. Appleton Century Crofts, Connecticut.

Eardley, A. (1992) Smear Campaign. *Health Serv. J.,* 29 August, pp. 28–29.

Eddy, D.M. & Eddy, J.F. (1984) Patient delay in the detection of cancer. *Proceedings of American Cancer Society, Fourth National Conference on Human Values and Cancer.* American Cancer Society, New York.

Elkind, A.K. (1981) The accuracy of nurses' knowledge about survival rates for early cancer in four sites. *J. of Adv. Nurs.* **6,** 35–40.

Elkind, A.K. (1982) Nurses' views about cancer. *J. of Adv. Nurs.,* **7,** 43–50.

Faulder, C. (1992) Breast awareness: What do we really mean? *Eur. J. of Cancer.* **28A** (10) 1595–6.

Forrest, P. (1986) *Breast Cancer Screening*. Report to the Health Ministers of England, Wales and Scotland and Northern Ireland. Her Majesty's Stationery Office, London.

Gowing, N. & Fisher, C. (1988) The General Pathology of Tumours. In *Oncology for Nurses and Health Care Professionals* (eds R. Tiffany & P. Pritchard) 2nd edn. Vol. 7. Harper & Row, Beaconsfield.

Holmes, P. (1987) Examining the Evidence. *Nursing Times.* **83** (31), 28–30.

MacGregor, J.E. *et al.* (1986) Cervical Cancer Screening in North East Scotland. In *Screening for Cancer of the Uterine Cervix.* (Eds M. Hakama, A.B. Miller, N. Day) 76, 25–36. IARC Scientific Publications, Lyons.

Macleod Clark, J.H., Haverty, S. & Kendall, S. (1989) Communication and Health Education in Nursing: Exploring the Nurse's Role in Helping Patients and Clients to Give Up Smoking. In *Directions in Nursing Research,* (Eds J. Wilson-Barnett & S. Robinson). Scutari, London.

Maguire, G.P., Lee, G.G., Bevington, D.J., Kinchermann, C.S., Crabtree, R.J. & Cornell, C.E. (1978) Psychiatric problems in the first year after mastectomy. *Brit. Med. J.* **1**, 963–5.

Maher, E. (1982) Anomic Aspects of Recovery from Cancer. *Social Science and Medicine*, **16**, 907–14.

McDonald, T.W., Neutens, J.J., Fischer, L.M. & Jessee, D. (1989) Impact of cervical intraepithelial neoplasia diagnosis and treatment on self-esteem and body image. *Gynaecologic Oncology.* **34**, 345–9.

McIntosh, J. (1974) Processes of communication, information seeking and control associated with cancer: a selective review of the literature. *Social Science and Medicine*, **8**, 167–87.

Meyskens, F.L. (1992) Strategies for Prevention of Cancer in Humans. *Oncology.* **6** (2) supplement, 15–24.

Posner, T. & Vessey, M. (1988) *Prevention of Cervical Cancer – the Patients' View.* King's Fund, London.

Pownall, M. (1986) News focus: the genital touch. *Nursing Times*, 12 February, 16–17.

Rowland, J.H. & Holland, J.C. (1989) Breast Cancer. In *Handbook of Psychooncology.* (eds J.C. Holland & J.H. Rowland) Oxford University Press, Oxford.

Sontag, S. (1979) *Illness as Metaphor.* Allen Lane, London.

Sontag, S. (1988) *Aids and its Metaphors.* Allen Lane, London.

Tross, S. & Holland, J.C. (1989) Psychological Sequelae in Cancer Survivors. In *Handbook of Psychooncology* (Eds J.C. Holland & J.H. Rowland) Oxford University Press, Oxford.

Weisman, A.D. & Worden, J.W. (1976) The existential plight in cancer, significance of the first 100 days. *Int. J. of Psychiatry in Med.*, **7**, (1) 1–15.

Chapter 13
Health Promotion and Nursing Practice

As a broad over-arching concept, health promotion can be seen as a philosophy which guides the way nurses and health carers should support and care for people. This book epitomizes this notion as health promotion values are used to explain and re-interpret priorities for the health service. Through a general process of encouraging consumerism, influence and participation from clients the service should become more relevant to needs, and less distant and impersonal and more fair in the way resources are distributed.

In order to reflect these goals, the ways nurses work and the way the care is given need to be scrutinized rigorously. So much of what we do pre-empts opportunities for discussion with patients, families or clients in many settings. In the past, patterns of care delivery may have become inflexible, routine and geared to slightly outmoded principles and values. In future, goals for nursing and the aims of health promotion should be the same. We should be working to improve, maintain or restore optimum levels of health – a complex and shared responsibility. Clearly, as shown by the preceding chapters, this can only be achieved with the collaboration of those we serve and work with. No longer can health care staff 'do things to people' with a clear conscience. Their action should be determined by what is decided with clients and also, at times, with their families. Prescription should give way to negotiation and all staff should realize that their contribution is only one small influence on health, satisfaction and welfare.

For too long nurses in the hospital setting have focused their attention on individuals, believing that this is most effective in improving the general level of health among the population. At times we have also included the family members in plans for care and future support at home. Of late, there is more realization that far more general factors influence the well-being and health of the general population. As the first chapters in this book so clearly state, nursing should be directed at those general policy issues as well as the individualized approach to care. By increasing awareness among staff of how social and physical environments affect styles of life, interactions and plans for care become more meaningful and staff can hopefully really offer good support for those in difficulty. Recognition of this global pattern of influences may lead to certain feelings of helplessness for us all, the challenge being too large, but the real future challenge is to be creative and innovative within the system and to be health oriented in all we do. Realistic appraisal is essential for success and the previous chapters translate the philosophy into action.

This concluding chapter aims to extract common themes for nurses from the preceding chapters to ensure we act as health promoting agents. In their choice of authors and topics the editors have purposefully chosen a broad range of specialties, client groups and settings. This reflects the variety of roles nurses can adopt but also demonstrates how a unifying approach or common philosophy to helping people is interpreted across different settings.

Shifting the balance of effort and resources

Prevention of much ill health is possible but this requires a shift in the balance of effort and resources away from the acute medical services towards a pro-active and supportive role for many health care workers. Nurses in particular have a part to play in this. That effort involves research to assess the most effective strategies for raising awareness and of modifying factors influencing health. It also requires motivation and confidence within our ranks to alter both professional approaches and organization of staff. The preceding chapters have demonstrated ways in which this may be done, both for those who are apparently healthy and for those at risk or suffering. They have also shown that there is much unnecessary sickness and many ways in which those in receipt of care could benefit more if this was more oriented to giving them real choice, directing their goals for care towards achieving adjustment, family support and positive self care.

Much of the work in this area reflects the basic needs for individuals to feel in control of their lives. Lack of such security can arise through inadequate resources – financial, personal, or social – and through illness and loss. The clear message underlying health promotion is to provide and organize such resources to enable people to cope. With more relevant information and more perceived close professional support many would not suffer or become vulnerable from fragmented and conflicting interventions. Although some authors use the term empowerment, achieving control over one's life and environment is synonymous with this and is more familiar to some disciplines of relevance to nursing.

In order to achieve this sense of control, staff must cease to assume they know best and must really attempt to understand and negotiate action which is chosen by the recipients. Not only individuals but the whole health care system should become consumer-oriented. The Patients' Charter (HMSO, 1992) should be cited endlessly where appropriate, as political will supported this consumerist notion. However, it may only be possible to encourage outspoken and knowledgeable consumers when staff are confident enough to cope with this themselves. Part of this confidence relies on developing a maturity and openness towards health issues. True commitment to health promotion may only be achieved when nurses and their colleagues not only understand the meaning of good health as the influential factor but internalize this to such an extent that this directs their personal and professional behaviour.

Positive mental health, clearly explained by Elizabeth Armstrong, occurs when demands and challenges are compatible with abilities and resources. Social support is often determined by mental status; when demands become over-taxing social support may not be provided and professional help may be required. For nurses it would be a great achievement to realize when demands or situations were becoming stressful and extra support was required. Greater self-awareness of both mental and physical health among staff could help them to be more sensitive to the needs of others and to the relevance of early support, preventing morbidity.

Through greater self-awareness and self-discovery, Project 2000 curricula are designed to promote confidence and a facility in nurses to provide healthy support or partnership in care. Hopefully students will have been treated as adults and will despise any form of interaction which would deny respect and full autonomy to clients. They should also have sufficient intellectual ability to analyse the health messages and discuss these with people who want to make choices. For example, as Jessica Corner suggests, decisions about screening are complex and not without some disadvantages, not the least being the cost of programmes. If nurses themselves decide on healthy options and appraise the options for screening they should not feel threatened by someone who adopts an alternative strategy by refusing screening opportunities.

Sadly it is necessary to reiterate this approach to education because until it is widespread and successful the true test of the therapeutic and positive effects on health care cannot be assessed. There is abundant evidence reviewed by David Sines for those with learning disability and by Jill Macleod Clark in health visiting and Sue Latter in acute care (cited in Chapter 5), that imposition of a paternalistic system of care is deter-

mined by previous models of education. In the past students have not
been treated as independent and responsible adults. Respect for oneself
is thought to lead to respect for others and from others. A true partnership with clients will only develop if this is based on self-determination and a belief that their wishes are pre-eminent. They thus have the
rights and choices to live their lives as independently as possible.

Partnership or true involvement by clients can also only be encouraged through an understanding of their viewpoint and situation. Providing holistic care may become a cliché but the editors of this book
clearly expound the view that mental, physical and social health are
interdependent. The split in nursing education between physical and
mental nursing has been based on the false premise of Descartes' dual-
istic philosophy which envisaged this dichotomy. 'Health nursing',
coined by Jill Macleod Clark, involves seeing the whole person and really
helping them to clarify their preferences and goals. Her research
demonstrates that smoking cessation is predicated on individual motivation to stop and support reinforcing this decision. Thus physical risk
can only be reduced through awareness of psychological processes.

Alleviating distress has always been a fundamental goal. Anxiety
associated with fears about health, worries about how a family member
will cope with a caring role and depression associated with bereavement, may all be examples where psychological reactions affect physical
health. Resources and skills must be developed among nurses to ensure
appropriate interventions. Different types of intervention for clearly
tailored information-giving, for empathic support during a home visit
and more thorough and continuous counselling may all be forms of
health promotion. This is necessary to reduce dysphonia or distressing
negative emotions but also is preventative in that further problems may
be allayed.

Public and community health

Most nursing has been targeted at individuals and some has been
directed at helping their families. Previously it was only the community
nursing services that attempted to assess and influence patterns of
health across communities. Some local and national programmes have
been aimed at promoting health awareness and policies have been
adopted to avoid endemic or poor general health. Dinah Gould explained
how national policies can directly affect individuals' health and how a
knowledge of infection spread may be curtailed by community-wide
action.

The shift towards reflecting community needs and towards building on the will and energy of individuals to work together for better health care is laudable. Self-help groups and locally-run facilities can be created in a way which reflects need sensitively. Dangers of professional dominance are avoided and evidence in this book attests to the sense of commitment and inherent benefits accruing from such active participation. Again it appears that control or empowerment to achieve a useful support mechanism is positive. Such a sense of responsibility arising from a clear identification of need is fundamental to health promotion.

When discussing community responsibility, David Sines reflected on the public's reaction to those with learning disabilities. Lack of understanding and the consequences of prejudice can be seen as negative or health decreasing. Given that social interaction is essential for so much of human existence, deprivation of this can be so destructive. Changing attitudes will probably take several generations but exemplary behaviour from nurses may serve to convince others that social stigma is intolerable.

Shifting from an individualistic to a more public orientation involves nurses recognizing the consequence of political forces and the dire consequences on health of a poor national economy. Facilities are reduced, and funding cuts in this country may result in few positive initiatives or even lead to inadequate provision for maintaining established services. Given the indubitable relationship between poverty and ill-health, professionals should use their abilities to convince others that health is important and can be improved through social and community programmes, not only by large institutionally-based medical services. Consensus on this throughout this book is encouraging.

Yet in terms of national policy, the battle on tobacco sales still continues. Directly linked to cardio-vascular and neoplastic disease, direct and passive smoking is probably one of the most harmful habits. Other drug taking is of course serious but not quite so prevalent. Action to ban smoking in public places is still controversial and the government resist imposing really heavy taxation. The sadness that cigarette smoking is more common in the more economically deprived groups serves to increase the challenge of undertaking the problem. Ultimately sensitive and careful campaigns to prevent youngsters smoking are considered essential. However, nurses should consider this a hopeless task if they themselves are not motivated to preserve their own good health and stay non-smokers themselves.

Social policy issues inevitably raise notions of social justice. Freedom of the individual and respect for fundamental rights underpin most public statements, such as the Patients' Charter. David Sines' analysis shows how far we fail when considering the vulnerable in society. Poorer countries also have a poorer record on human rights and this is not surprising given the inequalities which persist. Far from preserving the egalitarian democracy, economic stringencies may threaten the health of many but in particular those unable to represent themselves. Some children, and the mentally disabled among them, are inevitably threatened by the condition of others. In relatively affluent nations proper provision has come to be expected, but recent media exposés of the desperate plight of refugees and those dependent on institutional care demonstrate how political conflict can damage health and health care provision.

Collaboration

Just as health professionals should aim to influence politicians through reason and evidence, so should they attempt to influence each other. Such collaboration is essential for open and informed health care terms who understand the goals of health promotion. Correcting unhelpful paternalistic attitudes and encouraging an egalitarian and considerate mode of working is essential if health promotion is to flourish. Respect for individuals' feelings and autonomy has been emphasized throughout this text. It is impossible to work in an environment which does not reflect this, while at the same time attempting to ensure that all recipients of care are treated appropriately.

Nurses in particular have realized that health promotion reflects the ethos and values under primary nursing (or the new nursing). This has been explained in many papers but evidence for a research study carried out by King's College Department of Nursing Studies, cited by Jill Macleod Clark, demonstrated that it was only where primary nursing was established that health promotion was advanced. The confidence and value placed on individual nursing staff in their work by themselves and others was evident from interview and observation data. Much nurse-patient and nurse-relative intervention was focused on assessing and meeting the need for information and on future plans for care.

This type of progress is heartening. However, medical staff have been slow on many wards to accept that change is necessary and have been obstructive at times. This may hopefully only be a transitional problem and nurses themselves need to improve their ability to articulate the goals of primary nursing as well as the changes in ward organization necessary. Other team members must also accept such change and reflect the philosophy of negotiated and planned care with patients foremost in decision-making.

Teamwork should then be built around the clients' wishes. Progress in community care and family practice should now be emulated in acute settings. High technologically oriented care may be necessary at times but explicit values of really listening to patients and families and respecting their decisions are essential. The medically dominated intensive care unit may evoke anxiety; this combined with the life-threatening nature of the patient's condition should not permit staff to take decisions and exclude the family and patient.

Members of the public may be surprised at increased levels of consultation and negotiating in some acute care settings but early evidence from primary nursing units in particular suggest this is readily accepted. Yet family members can be encouraged even more to become involved in care, not from a standpoint that nurses are relinquishing responsibility but as appropriate and desired by such relatives. Effectively they do need to assess that this is valued by the patient.

Communication strategies

Throughout this book different forms of communication have been mentioned. From most media awareness campaigns to group work or formal or official documents, the way ideas are expressed is of vital importance. Clear communication in writing is essential and documents such as the Patients' Charter attempt to strike a balance between formality and ease of readership. However, reducing the seriousness of government publications by illustrating with pictures of 'little people' may be attractive but rather denigrating for the reader. Careful thought to such consequences is therefore important to avoid any suggestion of paternalism.

Several contributors to this book have discussed the style of face-to-face communication as central to health promotion. Jill Macleod Clark's work and that of Sally Kendall cited in Chapter 5 provide evidence that active listening, encouraging clients to identify aspects of their situation which may be harmful to their health, is fundamental to a health orientation. Only when individuals themselves manage to clarify their own thoughts and priorities can a health carer really start to support them through relevant information-giving and encouragement. Positive outcomes, such as smoking cessation, are found to be more likely with this style of interaction. Countless examples of imposition and prescription are found when nurse-patient interactions are analysed. Coining the phrase 'sick nursing' is useful in that it reflects an out-dated method of professional dominance, where the nurse decides what is done and blocks the real psychological work which needs to be undertaken by the recipient.

A constant challenge therefore presents itself to staff. Frequently learned tactics of dominating conversations and interrupting clients, patients or their family members, are hard to break. Asking open questions and following responses by probes ensures that topics or concerns are explored in depth. In contrast to the rapidly 'turning' and nurse-led interaction so frequently found, this provides opportunities for assessing worries and patient/client-led possibilities for resolutions.

This is akin to the counselling model employed in the psychiatric sphere, which employs a non-directive approach and aims to bring out the respondents' views and feelings about a situation. Emotional involvement with personal health risks or problems is seen to reflect commitment to change by Macleod Clark and others. Anxiety or even distress over issues may not appear initially helpful; nurses may even be blamed for upsetting their patients. In the longer term, however, this may well lead to positive behaviour change. Clearly though, it is essential to support an individual and their family at the time of painful recognitions such as acknowledged health risk and necessary change in lifestyle.

Changing behaviours

Although this may be an ultimate and ideal choice for some, it is problematic to hold rigid, professional views of what should be done when clients are not willing to accept these views. Nurses certainly need to follow through the principle of open choice for all as long as they feel confident that information and access to this has been facilitated for those for whom it is relevant. Old style paternalism would result if they became over-zealous in their attempts at persuasion that the healthy way was best.

Issues raised about the ethics of health promotion by Alan Cribb and Alison Dines and the success of screening for cancer by Jessica Corner are relevant to this. Autonomy and choice are of primary importance and integral to the idea of health promotion. Imposition of another's views thus becomes unacceptable, although they certainly have a right to be listened to. It is rare for this freedom to be denied in a health care setting but for the community at large this presents more of a dilemma. Smoking rates among teenagers are still increasing and research does not seem to indicate which are the most effective strategies to prevent this becoming a habit. Yet the conflict between free will and beneficence is apparent. Likewise screening for cancer (either breast or cervical) may only be truly effective with a 100% up-take. Surely there is enough uncertainty about the robustness and sensitivity of tests for all of us to question mass screening anyway. It may thus seem less obvious that a nurse has a clear remit to persuade women to comply with DoH advice. Her own views and analysis of data must also be respected.

Adopting generally healthy eating and exercise schedules is even less firmly established as a strategy to prevent morbidity. Geneticists are depressing in their confidence that the best way to live to a healthy old age is to choose the right parents! However there is evidence that obesity is closely linked with several physical problems. Encouraging behaviour change for those at risk of obesity (all of us) can therefore only take the form of an informative and positive conversation, exploring options and responses to these. For instance, patients who are post- myocardial often feel intensely relieved to be alive and desperate to avoid a repeat episode. Informed discussion on weight loss and smoking cessation is very appropriate and behaviour change may help individuals to feel they are in control of their lives, even if the evidence about prolongation of life is weak. However, primary prevention of myocardial infarction may be seen as more possible if USA figures can be extrapolated as in the last decade cardio-vascular death rates have started to decline. This may be associated with a greater health consciousness epitomized by runners in Fifth Avenue and an increase in vegetarian restaurants in the US cities.

Can we adopt health promotion in nursing?

By fostering progress from community action and really understanding the need for health promoting approaches to care, nurses could shift from a sickness (or sick role) orientation. By encouraging groups of people to take action and by raising the public's awareness of relevant issues, health carers could be far more influential at a social and political level. The divisions between political parties are relevant but given that continuous pressure and action is needed to improve health it is probably wise to influence all parties. At this national level nurses could be more effective, particularly on tobacco legislation and health care funding.

As Towell & Beardshaw's table, included in Chapter 8 indicates, various forms of involvement at all levels are called for. For instance, the notion of care packages for those with learning disability forms a really useful model of including community agents and others from health care facilities in co-operative ventures. These, in combination with voluntary and self-help groups, could form tremendously influential coalitions helping to inform and influence local policy. It is perhaps at the national and local level that early signs of progress are becoming evident. This should increase as Project 2000 qualified nurses will hopefully share this wider perspective on health promotion.

Even more challenging is the aim to reorientate the philosophy of hospital nursing to become more health promoting. Through careful reflection and analysis of opportunities to involve patients and families in health care, a greater assertion of their choices should be possible. This requires good role models and diligent support to constantly reinforce assertive communication skills among staff and open truly interactive supportive help for patients. Senior staff determine the atmosphere and 'culture' of wards and need to share successes and difficulties with each other when changing attitudes. Network support is vital for such change agents. Devoting time to psychological care and information exchange in the acute setting is essential for sensitive care planning. This can also provide a sound basis for a better standard of life at home after hospital discharge.

Family support still needs to be given a higher priority. Relative participation is rarely encouraged in acute adult settings, yet when it is welcomed or established positive outcome results. More confidence for relatives in managing at home certainly serves to promote adjustment to inevitable longer-term problems and leads to maximal independence or self-care abilities, as reviews of patient education research show. Despite these findings practice seems to lag behind, especially in non-specialist acute wards. However, if nurses on cardiac wards can manage to orientate this care to life beyond the ward, surely generalists can also do this.

Positive signs of democratization and truly patient-centred or patient-determined decisions are emerging. These are slow but this is not surprising in view of the radical shift in philosophy that this has involved for some. The health culture must involve all carers, but because of its impact and size the nursing profession as a group must exemplify this approach by learning skills and applying knowledge in ways which are sensitively tailored to those who need our care and support in the community and in hospital.

Reference

HMSO (1992). *The Patients' Charter: A Charter for Health.* Her Majesty's Stationery Office, London.

Appendix
Ottawa Charter for Health Promotion

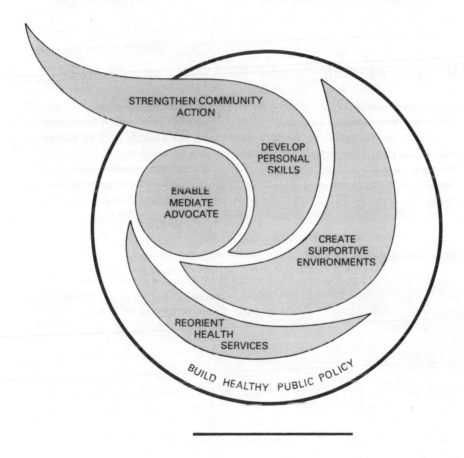

STRENGTHEN COMMUNITY ACTION

DEVELOP PERSONAL SKILLS

ENABLE MEDIATE ADVOCATE

CREATE SUPPORTIVE ENVIRONMENTS

REORIENT HEALTH SERVICES

BUILD HEALTHY PUBLIC POLICY

AN INTERNATIONAL CONFERENCE
ON HEALTH PROMOTION
The move towards a new public health

November 17–21, 1986, Ottawa, Ontario, Canada

CHARTER

The first International Conference on Health Promotion, meeting in Ottawa this 21st day of November 1986, hereby presents this Charter for action to achieve Health for All by the year 2000 and beyond.

This conference was primarily a response to growing expectations for a new public health movement around the world. Discussions focused on the needs in industrialized countries, but took into account similar concerns in all other regions. It built on the progress made through the Declaration on Primary Health Care at Alma Ata, the World Health Organization's Targets for Health for All document, and the recent debate at the World Health Assembly on intersectoral action for health.

Health promotion

Health promotion is the process of enabling people to increase control over, and to improve, their health. To reach a state of complete physical, mental and social well-being, an individual or group must be able to identify and to realize aspirations, to satisfy needs, and to change or cope with the environment. Health is, therefore, seen as a resource for everyday life, not the objective of living. Health is a positive concept emphasizing social and personal resources, as well as physical capacities. Therefore, health promotion is not just the responsibility of the health sector, but goes beyond healthy life-styles to well-being.

Prerequisites for health

The fundamental conditions and resources for health are peace, shelter, education, food, income, a stable eco-system, sustainable resources, social justice and equity. Improvement in health requires a secure foundation in these basic prerequisites.

Advocate

Good health is a major resource for social, economic and personal development and an important dimension of quality of life. Political, economic, social, cultural, environmental, behavioural and biological factors can all favour health or be harmful to it. Health promotion action aims at making these conditions favourable through *advocacy* for health.

Enable

Health promotion focuses on achieving equity in health. Health promotion action aims at reducing differences in current health status and ensuring equal opportunities and resources to *enable* all people to achieve their fullest health potential. This inclues a secure foundation in a supportive environment, access to information, life skills and opportunities for making healthy choices. People cannot achieve their fullest health potential unless they are able to take control of those things which determine their health. This must apply equally to women and men.

Mediate

The prerequisites and prospects for health cannot be ensured by the health sector alone. More importantly, health promotion demands coordinated action by all concerned: by governments, by health and other social and economic sectors, by non-governmental and voluntary organizations, by local authorities, by industry and by the media. People in all walks of life are involved as individuals, families and communities. Professional and social groups and health personnel have a major responsibility to mediate between differing interests in society for the pursuit of health.

Health promotion strategies and programmes should be adapted to the local needs and possibilities of individual countries and regions to take into account differing social, cultural and economic systems.

Health promotion action means:

Build healthy public policy

Health promotion goes beyond health care. It puts health on the agenda of policy makers in all sectors and at all levels, directing them to be aware of the health consequences of their decisions and to accept their responsibilites for health.

Health promotion policy combines diverse but complementary approaches including legislation, fiscal measures, taxation and organizational change. It is coordinated action that leads to health, income and social policies that foster greater equity. Joint action contributes to ensuring safer and healthier goods and services, healthier public services, and cleaner, more enjoyable environments.

Health promotion policy requires the identification of obstacles to the adoption of healthy public policies in non-health sectors, and ways of removing them. The aim must be to make the healthier choice the easier choice for policy makers as well.

Create supportive environments

Our societies are complex and interrelated. Health cannot be separated from other goals. The inextricable links between people and their environment constitute the basis for a socio-ecological approach to health. The overall guiding principle for the world, nations, regions and communities alike, is the need to encourage reciprocal maintenance – to take care of each other, our communities and our natural environment. The conservation of natural resources throughout the world should be emphasized as a global responsibility.

Changing patterns of life, work and leisure have a significant impact on health. Work and leisure should be a source of health for people. The way society organizes work should help create a healthy society. Health promotion generates living and working conditions that are safe, stimulating, satisfying and enjoyable.

Systematic assessment of the health impact of a rapidly changing environment – particularly in areas of technology, work, energy production and urbanization – is essential and must be followed by action to ensure positive benefit to the health of the public. The protection of the natural and built environments and the conservation of natural resources must be addressed in any health promotion strategy.

Strengthen community action

Health promotion works through concrete and effective community action in setting priorities, making decisions, planning strategies and implementing them to achieve better health. At the heart of this process is the empowerment of communities, their ownership and control of their own endeavours and destinies.

Community development draws on existing human and material resources in the community to enhance self-help and social support, and to develop flexible systems for strengthening public participation and direction of health matters. This requires full and continuous access to information, learning opportunities for health, as well as funding support.

Develop personal skills

Health promotion supports personal and social development through providing information, education for health and enhancing life skills. By so doing, it increases the options available to people to exercise more control over their own health and over their environments, and to make choices conducive to health.

Enabling people to learn throughout life, to prepare themselves for all of its stages and to cope with chronic illness and injuries is essential. This has to be facilitated in school, home, work and community settings. Action is required through educational, professional, commercial and voluntary bodies, and within the institutions themselves.

Reorient health services

The responsibility for health promotion in health services is shared among individuals, community groups, health professionals, health service institutions and governments. They must work together towards a health care system which contributes to the pursuit of health.

The role of the health sector must move increasingly in a health promotion direction, beyond its responsibility for providing clinical and curative services.

Health services need to embrace an expanded mandate which is sensitive and respects cultural needs. This mandate should support the needs of individuals and communities for a healthier life, and open channels between the health sector and broader social, political, economic and physical environmental components.

Reorienting health services also requires stronger attention to health research as well as changes in professional education and training. This must lead to a change of attitude and organization of health services, which refocuses on the total needs of the individual as a whole person.

Moving into the future

Health is created and lived by people within the settings of their everyday life; where they learn, work, play and love. Health is created by caring for oneself and others, by being able to take decisions and have control over one's life circumstances, and by ensuring that the society one lives in creates conditions that allow the attainment of health by all its members.

Caring, holism and ecology are essential issues in developing strategies for health promotion. Therefore, those involved should take as a guiding principle that, in each phase of planning, implementation and evaluation of health promotion activities, women and men should become equal partners.

Commitment to health promotion

The participants in this conference pledge:

- to move into the arena of healthy public policy, and to advocate a clear political commitment to health and equity in all sectors;
- to counteract the pressures towards harmful products, resource depletion, unhealthy living conditions and environments, and bad nutrition; and to focus attention on public health issues such as pollution, occupational hazards, housing and settlements.
- to respond to the health gap within and between societies, and to take the inequities in health produced by the rules and practices of these societies;
- to acknowledge people as the main health resource; to support and enable them to keep themselves, their families and friends healthy through financial and other means, and to accept the community as the essential voice in matters of its health, living conditions and well-being.
- to reorient health services and their resources towards the promotion of health; and to share power with other sectors, other disciplines and most importantly with people themselves.
- to recognize health and its maintenance as a major social investment and challenge; and to address the overall ecological issue of our ways of living.

The conference urges all concerned to join them in their commitment to a strong public health alliance.

Call for international action

The Conference calls on the World Health Organization and other international organizations to advocate the promotion of health in all appropriate forums and to support countries in setting up strategies and programmes for health promotion.

The Conference is firmly convinced that if people in all walks of life, non-governmental and voluntary organizations, governments, the World Health Organization and all other bodies concerned join forces in introducing strategies for health promotion, in line with the moral and social values that form the basis of this Charter, Health For All by the year 2000 will become a reality.

This Charter for action was developed and adopted by an international conference, jointly organized by the World Health Organization, Health and Welfare Canada and the Canadian Public Health Association. Two hundred and twelve participants from 38 countries met from 17 to 21 November, 1986, in Ottawa, Canada to exchange experiences and share knowledge of health promotion.

The Conference stimulated an open dialogue among lay, health and other professional workers, among representatives of governmental, voluntary and community organizations, and among politicians, administrators, academics and practitioners. Participants coordinated their efforts and came to a clearer definition of the major challenges ahead. They strengthened their individual and collective commitment to the common goal of Health for All by the Year 2000.

This Charter for action reflects the spirit of earlier public charters through which the needs of people were recognized and acted upon. The Charter presents fundamental strategies and approaches for health promotion which the participants considered vital for major progress. The Conference report develops the issues raised, gives concrete examples and practical suggestions regarding how real advances can be achieved, and outlines the action required of countries and relevant groups.

The move towards a new public health is now evident worldwide. This was reaffirmed not only by the experiences but by the pledges of Conference participants who were invited as individuals on the basis of their expertise. The following countries were represented: Antigua, Australia, Austria, Belgium, Bulgaria, Canada, Czechoslovakia, Denmark, Eire, England, Finland, France, German Demoncratic Republic, Federal Republic of Germany, Ghana, Hungary, Iceland, Israel, Italy, Japan, Malta, Netherlands, New Zealand, Northern Ireland, Norway, Poland, Portugal, Romania, St. Kitts-Nevis, Scotland, Spain, Sudan, Sweden, Switzerland, Union of Soviet Socialist Republics, United States of America, Wales and Yugoslavia.

Index